HIV, Mon Amour

The James Laughlin Award is given to commend and support a poet's second book. The only award of its kind in the United States, it is named in honor of the poet and publisher James Laughlin (1914–1997), who founded New Directions in 1936. The award is endowed by a gift to The Academy of American Poets from the Drue Heinz Trust.

The publication of this book was supported by a grant from the Eric Mathieu King Fund of The Academy of American Poets.

HIV, Mon Amour

Poems

Tory Dent

The Sheep Meadow Press
Riverdale-on-Hudson, New York

Copyright © 1999 by Tory Dent

All inquiries and permission requests should be addressed to:
The Sheep Meadow Press
PO Box 1345
Riverdale-on-Hudson, NY 10471

Cover: Andy Warhol, *Big Electric Chair*, 1967. Centre Georges Pompidou

Designed and typeset by Sheep Meadow Press
Photograph by Arne Svenson
Distributed by University Press of New England

Printed on acid-free paper in the United States. This book meets the guidelines for permanence and durability of the Committee on Production Guidelines for Book Longevity of the Council on Library Resources.

Library of Congress Cataloging-in-Publication Data:

Dent, Tory, 1958-
     HIV, Mon Amour / Tory Dent
                    p.   cm.
          ISBN 1-878818-81-3 (acid-free paper)
          I. HIV-positive women--Poetry. I. Title.
          PS3554.E586 H58 1999   99-046988
          8111.54--dc21   CIP

          ISBN 1-878818-86-4 (acid-free paper)

Dying means: you are dead already, in an immemorial past, of a death which was not yours, which you have thus neither known nor lived, but under the threat of which you believe you are called upon to live; you await it henceforth in the future, constructing a future to make it possible at last— possible as something that will take place and will belong to the realm of experience.

Maurice Blanchot, *The Writing of the Disaster*

for Sean

Acknowledgments

"What Calendars Have Become" has been published in *American Poetry Review*.

"Family Romance" has been published in *The Kenyon Review*.

"Clash" has been published in *The Exact Change Yearbook*, edited
by Peter Gizzi.

"Make Costly Your Tears" has been published in *Agni* magazine.

"Everybody Loves a Winner" and "Voice as Gym-Body" have been
published in *Ploughshares*, guest editor Marilyn Hacker.

"The Crying Game" has been published in *Columbia: A Magazine
of Poetry & Prose*.

Stanzas "XIX," "XXI," "XXV," and "XXIX" from the long poem "HIV, Mon Amour"
have been published in *Pequod* as well as "XVII," "XIV," "X," "VII," and "II"
in my book of poems *What Silence Equals* (Persea Books), and "IV," "V," "XII," and "XX"
in *The World* under the title "*from* A Two Way Mirror."

"Future Text Panel" has been published in *Mudfish Magazine*.

"Omen" has been published in *Pataphysics*.

Stanza "XXXV" from "HIV, Mon Amour" was exhibited in "The Return of the
Cadavre Exquis" at the Drawing Center, New York City.

I would like to thank the New York Foundation for the Arts, Money for Women/Barbara
Deming Memorial Fund, the Rona Jaffe Foundation Writer's Award, and PEN Grants for
Writers with AIDS for their financial support. In addition I would like to express grati-
tude to the MacDowell Colony for the gift of time and privacy.

T.D.

Contents

I.

The Pressure

Fourteen Days in Quarantine

1.

The TB room posits itself as at once outside me like a Richard Serra,
contained, abstract as the scientific premise upon which it was founded,
while the 75 square feet and the ceiling vent, which circulates fresh air
every eight minutes, best represent my sense of interiority by virtue
of the falsification of representation. My reflection viewed in blankness,
the extra-large TV bolted too high up against the opposite wall (pale lime),
square box askew as if the quizzical head of some surveillance authority,
refuses to echo back what signifies reality to me. Instead I'm forced
to witness my own participation in the clinical process, a kind of snuff film
culturally condoned: I regard the woman illuminated by overhead fluorescence,
her features diminished as if rubbed away, clay bust banished to raw status,
her physical proportions distorted, more, then less with flame-like metamorphoses,
hooked up to an IV; O artificial extension of the body now commenced,
the transplantation of anatomized topography upon its badly damaged origin.
Hospital gown worn backwards, thus open at the neck, and I think what a great
Nan Goldin portrait it would make — "Tory, New York Hospital, January 1996."

2.

When they wheeled me up from ER into respiratory isolation the space radiated
as if a magnifying glass were put to it under a sunray. The afternoon sun
from the southern exposure hit interrogationally against my head,
efficacious as the chemotherapy drugs to which I'd become allergic,
my torso scalding red from the eventual conflation of the hives. I writhed
like an eel from the remote-control reconfiguring of my hospital bed, the way
diagrams of Hatha yoga postures present themselves on a page, Muybridge
stills repeated into the illusion of motion; I tried any position that might
ease the poltergeist-like progression of the "launched" reaction, unpredictable
in its phases. The days succeeded then in a condensed formula of alternate
darkness and light that make up twenty-four hours as I waited for my medication,
a dose every three hours: Benadryl, prednisone, shots of epinephrine, Atarax
while the room reverberated a cryptic quiet, my bygone and would-be world
held in abeyance beyond the gridded glass, where I in an incubated state of sorts
watched with voyeurist intensity the heads that only in profile would pass.

But the view out my window was fabulous. Not just a river view but
a long view of the East River which resembled the Thames, the Fifty-ninth Street
Bridge foregrounding its tranquil perfection, tugboats and flatliners
moving out and upstream like alligators with only the most moderate ripples
made in the water. The world was gracefully, and thus almost archaically,
silenced behind the double-cased window, like a *film noir* short or
Stieglitz's New York. It was as if the city itself, in solidarity with my life,
stopped and paused, as a gesture of respect, a tactful response for a long,
two-week moment so that I could reassess, positioning one of the three chairs
in my room dead center before it where ceremoniously I developed the habit
of taking my breakfast, while Schubert or Kiri Te Kanawa played not so softly
on my black boombox. Later, when the pentamidine pulsated through my body,
which grew weaker and more tired until I receded in sync with the daylight
from chair back to bed as if falling backwards in slow motion, the way
a display dummy does during a rehearsed car crash, the river, though enveloped
in fog and pollution, remained, blurred line detected through cracked shield,
and gave an impression of the infinite: the possibility of my getting out
of there, of living perhaps, even thirty more years as once I had expected.

The night sky would hang aloof and autonomous as a piece of Fabergé jewelry,
an example of Dionysiac craftsmanship that no longer pertained to my century.
The uplit skyscrapers of some famous buildings, Chrysler, Citicorp, amidst
residential and business, the windows alternately dark or filled with bright
coldness, introduced, like ink spilled on virgin paper, a kind of filmy,
alternate-state wattage from which one could expect the birth of something;
some transgression of physical properties, some otherworldly entity, gooey and
fetus-faced, reaching out to me only. But only a pattern, arbitrary, absolute
of lights, lonely and tiny, lay out against the lawless expansion, a game
of dominos played cursorily in the hawking blankness, bipartisan, yes,
in its PC chaos but neglectful and rancorous in this fail-safe,
do-no-harm schematic: the more godless the landscape, the more demonically
driven the agenda. Bored by ideas of persecution and fatigued with my efforts
to connect sign with meaning, closure, and hence beginning, I turn my head,
heavy and mechanical, pull the strangulating cord to turn off the overhead
fluorescence, and allow what balance this queer harmony of weakness and strength
might make, the pallor of city lights lending an alien glow to my limbs.
I glance at the night sky then back to the TV void, trying to distinguish natural

from man-made in order to identify that with which I identify. The treatment,
a chemical, incites cell renewal by virtue of the body's ability to synthetically
substitute itself: icon upon ideal. Think of it as restoration, I say out loud.

5.

There was a single piece of art in the room, good art too, if you can believe it.
It was a photograph, black and white, of a landscape taken in the Southwest,
somewhere arid, where the sky outruns the desert, a cowboy's idea of finisterre.
It hung straight ahead like a crucifix from the upright-positioned stare
I would motor into prolonged spectatorship that served, I guess, in lieu of prayer.
The image was of a flat-topped mountain indigenous to Utah or Wyoming, its profile,
which threw into high relief the parched, plebeian horizon, exhibited a staggered
growth of progress and sharp decline like the invisible statistic charts held up
prototypically before me, black mourning veils that obscure my perception
of what could be otherwise. But the predicted deterioration of my body delineated
against the amorphous space of possibility was not so unlike the mountain's outline.
Its earthen form, hulking and ancient, could be read as in ruins or unstoppable
despite past corrections. Regardless, it prevailed if only in idea as appropriated
by the photograph, calling into question the category of "origin", mine in particular.
Where exactly have been set the perimeters between my body and the self that exists
outside my consciousness? In the little synaptic connections when people think of me?
Or in postcards and outdated e-mails reread in the aftermath of my scientific death,
different from the cultural death, the emotional death, the spiritual death;
different from a sea burial, from the char and ash and bone and fabric devoured
by the Atlantic, swallowed, digested and spat out again, generic as saline liquid?

6.

I was almost never alone. For someone quarantined this seemed strange to me.
Aside from visitors there were nurses, technicians, and attending doctors in addition
to my physician, as well as residents and interns who woke me at six in small groups,
poking, thumping, and speaking too loudly. There were hospital workers of every
division: the food bearer, the floor washer, the temperature/blood pressure taker,
the sheet changers who stripped and made my bed with military exactness as I
listened to the crisp, unnerving sounds of starched cotton pulled to uniform
precision. Often several people came at once, or in short succession, wearing masks,
of course, morphed into bodies with just eyes, their monkey jaw disguises shifting in
adjustment. It was theater, either Ionescian, in which the IV poles & pumps, buckets &
mops, EKG machines entered like a procession of bizarre animals; or Artaudian, where
I, both audience and stage, served as witness of exequy and its nexus, the centripetal

force commissioning event. When a rare moment of solitude would descend, billowing, augmented by the white noise of the fresh-air vent that upheld the rigors of Health Dept. standards, it invariably threw me, never getting used to this terroristic aspect of pleasurable tease before unexpected assault. Once I opted not to seize the chance to close my eyes or piss in private, and walked instead, cautiously, to the door. Peering out the gridded glass at the junglesque activity of the hospital corridor, I saw their full faces so different than imagined from the partial viewing previously presented like progressional sketches of a criminal. One nurse noticed me mesmerized by this game of identification and scowled in discouragement until I recoiled. Watching was interpreted as an act of taunting, the behavior of mental patients or prisoners; an interpretation that was, in turn, a defense for their guilt, for the sympathy they as professionals, in order to perform well, could not allow. They knew what my watching really meant: the longing to be healthy, to be like them.

7.

In the beginning I tried to write. I would define the beginning as that brief interval between the subsiding of the allergic reaction and the reintroduction of the TB drugs, before the full force of the daily pentamidine was felt. During this window of time, less than forty-eight hours, I was "myself" again like the child prostitute interviewed on A&E who now, as herself, is a happy, young mother. Her name is Nina. She was abducted at 12 years of age. She recuperates the particularly harrowing account of when she disappeared from the street, some pimp she had been sold to at a discount for aging to 17, locking her in the basement of his dilapidated ranch house, normal protocol for the modern slave master. He shot her up with heroin when he was sick of her and made her sleep. Then he shot her up with coke when he needed some cash to retool his alcohol habit. She survived this way for three years before she was found. I am watching her narration (not a confession because there has been no wrongdoing) from my hospital bed. Free cable is one of many perks on the AIDS floor. I open up my laptop inspired by how I perversely identify with her, my body, sweet, pale thing, kidnapped also in a way; my legs, with their muscles atrophied, have completely changed shape, all bruise-dotted up from syringes. I let one dangle, engaged fishing pole, over the edge, assuming the perpendicular position of concentration I know. I touch the keyboard. The cold plastic alphabet singes, strangely forbidden, therefore erotic. I realize slowly, as if in orgasmic stages of cunnilingus, that the most elementary effort of extending toward the familiar, of taking control of my body, of pushing out articulations, has become transgressive; as perhaps it became to Nina, in between highs, when experiencing "herself" for a single minute, she risked investigation of the padlocked cellar door.

During my hospitalization, the great blizzard of '96 occurred, devastating the Tri-State areas and delaying my dinner. My view holed up like the porthole of an igloo, crystalline and anesthetized. Loyal visitors arrived at odd hours like Pa gone to town in *The Little House on the Prairie*, shaking off the snow on their coats, perspiring a bit amidst the sudden warmth of the room, their glow in high contrast with the matte temperancy of the quarantine masks. My experience of the storm was limited to this internality of it, something of what a fetus records of the wide world while in the womb, watching CNN coverage for visuals: shivering newscasters shouting their emphases, cars stalled in zigzag procession, inter-mittent shots of portly snowplows saving the day. It seemed like fun. Remarkably to me I remain in respiratory confinement as everybody flays about, hospital shifts contorted, nurses forced to perform a technician's duties, doctors stooped to pulse taking. I watch all the flutter as if through convex glass, atypical viewer trapped in a 60's Arrid Extra Dry commercial: noses loom large and spectacled eyes hysterically wide. I witness as a separatist, as caged animals do the weirdos on the other side of the wire who experiment upon them. I regard the snow and the snowstorm extravaganza at arm's length, a great, hairy hand collaring me in the effort to inject or extract some substance. I am purposely held away from the element, in part discriminatorily, but also, by virtue of this pejorative intent, the way last comes first in Christian ethics, as if having risen above it, ether-like as steam did climb nefariously off the river, immune to cold, indifferent to the wetness, blanched to the color white, and how I once loved it for I'd become it, the other, the terrifying, the nuance, the inhuman.

9.

I knew that one day I might look back at this interval as when I was better off, as when the room was private, as when drugs were considered useful, as a time when I could sit up, as a time when I could argue. I knew that especially at night after 2 in the morning when my third dose of the allergic reaction protocol had just been administered, prednisone & Atarax (the Benadryl had been worthless) followed by a shot of epinephrine stinging me into intergalactic awakeness, the stages of bodily absorption, shivering, tingling, sudden dumb calm and subsequent relief from the physical screaming, I would monitor mentally with the hope of willing the response into actuality later, when the drug would be refused to me; when I knew I had been better off tolerating another prick of the needle. The nurse pulls the string switching off the overhead fluorescence, the click rudely loud, the plastic pulls snapping back against my face for a second. I experience a memory flash of the moment before — the sound

of Velcro from the blood pressure cuff, the little white pill-dispensing cups,
her cold fingertips on my pulse, the beautiful syringe poised impressively
between her teeth as she read her watch. Lying down on my side in the
quickening darkness, my position unchanged from when I received the injection,
I watch through the hospital bed guard rail as she leaves, the stillborn silence
of my room undisturbed save for the squeak of her white shoes on the freshly
cleaned floor, and the whoosh of the heavy quarantine door automatically closing.
A brief flooding of corridor light appears on the linoleum tiles, then nothing.

10.

My physician arrived every day at about 9:00 am, announcing himself with that jingle
of raps on my door which signifies a friend, not foe, outside. He never
wore the prerequisite quarantine mask, perhaps because he knew the perimeters
of exposure and didn't feel his short visits to be a danger or perhaps because
he thought that communicating with a full face was important for our discussions,
for my confidence in him, in the treatment decisions, in myself as something
more than another verified statistic with tubes flowing out from my
limbs attached to plastic bags of clear medication, my form reconfigured as
needing something larger than a god, something scientifically derived in order
to be sustained. For the most part it worked, the matching up of my two identities,
the reality of me sick and the memory of me well, centered my soul like glass
slides containing a blood smear for microscopic inspection. Particularly in the eye
contact when we discussed the alternatives, in the pauses after when we remained
looking at each other in mutual contemplation of the seriousness of the situation,
I would sense myself positioned thus between the imagined researcher's hands.
And the gut feeling I had always associated with the word "Tory", the specific
white pine amidst the general landscape, would be brought into sharp focus as if
gently held down, trembling vase on rudimentary table within the bomb shelter
security of the room. We would watch almost as if a third party were present,
the potential for it to be blown apart like any ordinary structure in a tornado,
where wooden fences lie prostrate and barn animals soar upward into an ever obscuring
sky; where I, a juxtapositional series of flashbacks and idiosyncratic urges
superimposed upon each other like pages of a memoir that comprises a kinetic, almost
moaning kind of narrative, might disappear also into the indefeasible spiral above.

11.

On the eve before the TB drugs were reintroduced, my physician and I
tossed a coin in order to decide which one would likely cause another
allergic response akin to that which had required hospitalization a week

earlier. The embossed profile of George Washington signified rifampin instead
of isoniazid, a choice that brought no reassurance since the outcome remained
equally uncertain: I continued revolving, a quarter dollar in the air, glints
of fluorescence ricocheting off our forefather's cheekbone, the claw-foot of
the eagle alighted atop of neither branch nor rock. I beheld, beholden to the
sight as if some mystical vision, the literal turning of my fate, its infinite
axis where, like a glistened pig self-reflecting on the spit, or a convertible
that, having overshot its ultimate goal of the highway, teeters upon a
cracked precipice, I lay as if held out, a barbaric gift. A slab of marble
was the gurney cot of my hospital bed and the springs digging against my back
could be interrupted as actual pressure from the vast, the pale, from the
frameless filigree of winter branches, skyscrapers, and truncated river. To
that from which no voice would emit I was forced to entrust my failing body
my life's possessions in a bundle and stick, willed to their abandonment.
It seemed as if the days and nights I spent in quarantine evolved into a
kind of extension of that eve, that particular night a metonymical event
occurring within the greater overarching eve that delineates this world
from the next, the schematic of which one experiences as sinking into twilight
the way the shipwrecked do into the ocean, the way HIV overrides my body as
if overwriting the flesh, the waterline rising above my upturned, gasping face.
It was as if my body were asking for the privilege to be viewed as remains,
to be given the opportunity to float unfettered away from me, to struggle
for a while, alternately bob and drown, allowed to live or die on its own.

12.

My boyfriend arrived straight from work every night at 6:30 pm, his smiling
face displayed momentarily in the square of gridded glass like puppet theater
before he entered donning his quarantine mask. Often he brought the something
I had requested, articles which covered a spectrum of needs, acting as conduit
to the outside world through which, what was life proper compared to this,
made itself available to me: flowers, cassette tapes, favorite home items
such as my pillow or bedside lamp or cosmetic oddity with the unpronounceable
brand name, special foods divergent from the hospital menu heated in the
nurses' canteen microwave. Sometimes these secular pleasures had to be coaxed
as when I had no appetite and sat in upright confrontation with my bowl of
homemade minestrone, head turned left then right, any position to avoid the fumes
while he pleaded, even argued. But the pleasure of touch I never refused when he
climbed gently into the narrow cot with me, winter jacket still on, the sudden
cold of his earlobes against my cheek, the thick cardboard material of the
quarantine mask which we would defiantly indent in order to kiss. Our eyes

would stay open staring into the other's pupil until practically cross-eyed.
The last thing we wanted was more mystery, more left to the imagination. Only
what was before us now would satisfy. It was as if all our sexual experiences
individual and combined, came to closure in this exchange, exposing themselves
as spoiled representations of erotic desire. That base instinct belonging to
animal of muscle, semen, bone, raw appetite, we perceived in retrospect as
mannered like ballroom dance, misguided in topical obsession, over-fucked until
it fell outside the realm of its origin. Erogenous zones are beside the point.
It's the eye, the voice disguised as organ and orifice, that penetrates and receives.

13.

I lay upon the recesses of sheets in the darkness, the gradations of black
and white, of light and obscurity, artificial and natural passing over me like
prehistoric birds, their giant and frightening feathered wings obstructing the
sun then not. I lay there like would-be carrion on sand dune and sea grass while
they flew overhead, my hair incrementally disturbed by the smallest breeze their
flapping incurred. Their shrieks exchanged resonated as faraway but knife-precise
in the ability to disturb me. Everything hurt me. Day four into the allergic
reaction and the hives, enormous red welts that proliferated like weeds or
red ants all over my body, swelling my eyes shut, closing my throat, finally
subsided in progression, the next stage of my body's rejection of itself, their
confluence into skin burning crimson as if the workings of the world had reversed
from exterior to interior operation, where ultraviolet rays blazed forcefully
from inside me. What's most terrifying about sickness is its fascist self-
containment, the seizing of the body by itself, the warring efforts toward
redemption of selfhood and its defilement, the defeat produced by somatic betrayal.
The ally of my anatomy could no longer be trusted. I thought I was more than
a display of carnage though I'm still sentimentally attached to it as if to
a person rather than a decoy; like Freud's account of the *fort* (gone) *da* (here)
game in which a little boy plays hide-and-seek with a spool of thread that's
become the mother-substitute, compensating for his sense of abandonment. He
stages her disappearance in order to rehearse the pleasure of her return. Similarly,
I wish I could bury me myself the way Esther did her rag doll in *Bleak House*,
in the spirit of *fort* / *da*, then death could be welcomed as life's prelude.

I left the quarantine room three times. The first being the fruits of my successful manipulation of a nurse whom, toward the evening of day three, I begged to take me out. Initially my request made her uneasy, unable to maintain eye contact with me, busying herself with flushing my IV and reading my pulse. I made my plea incessant yet irresistible, the effort focused solely on the human connection, with ample articulation of her name and the magic word "please", my voice low and sweet, relatively calm. I hardly took a breath. Mention of my gratitude was made often as well as the promise that just a minute would suffice, the assurance that no one would notice, and that her general kindness would be praised to Patient Services. Then she stared at me and agreed. I wore a special blue TB mask different from the ones my visitors had to wear as we walked arm-in-arm like European girlfriends to the newly refurbished atrium where a man with KS slept upright in front of TV glare. We made stilted, self-consciously banal comments about the lights on the Fifty-ninth Street Bridge for five minutes then turned around. The second time was when I was wheeled to x-ray, the orderly alerting those ahead with his walkie-talkie that a TB patient was on her way so that rooms could be cleared and sealed off one by one as I rode through them. People forced to share the elevator with me glanced down at my masked and gowned figure with pity for the vermin level to which I had descended though they stood at a wide angle around me. The third time was my release, when I wore civilian clothes again, the blue jeans scratchy and stiff, my legs weak and unsteady but exhilarated by the whisking sound of walking out of quarantine, off the AIDS floor, out of the hospital and into the moist, gray January afternoon where the drizzle hit my face, cold and sharp, and the asphalt underfoot registered as especially hard.

Future Text Panel

in memory of Andrea Fisher

A fire going is the only sound
of my old life shrinking on the left with the sun.

The treetops, prolific as the sky, hide the sky.

My blood unnerves me.

The evidence of friends exists only in memory,
as if they were dead or as if I were dead,
my spirit slithering throughout the earth,
perhaps seeking revenge,
or in search of the deed I need to complete
to finally leave my body in peace
like a personage.
Bound to the unfinished,
silt still spills upon my grave,
upon my name engraved
I must wear in my exodus like Houdini's chains.

Voice as Gym-Body

for Marilyn Hacker

In order for a rapprochement with the physical body
Only necromancy could be behind it.
Racked on a stretcher the IV tubes string me up
Like a cello without a player.

Only necromancy could be behind it.
These days of horse-drawn betrayal.
Like a cello without a player
I'm caught, a crown of thorns, in a winter orchard.

These days of horse-drawn betrayal.
Impromptu night: tar ridge.
I'm caught, a crown of thorns, in a winter orchard,
A keyboard silent as the keyboard to deaf Beethoven.

Impromptu night: tar ridge.
I insert the child's hand literally into my chest,
A keyboard silent as the keyboard to deaf Beethoven.
As if a surgeon's, I warm it.

I insert the child's hand literally into my chest.
Fingers twitch like an impulse, final and emotive
As if a surgeon's, I warm it
With my voice (overbuilt to compensate for no child).

Fingers twitch like an impulse, final and emotive.
The way one man survived was by altarpiece commissions.
With my voice (overbuilt to compensate for no child)
Like an altarpiece, I try continually to build.

The way one man survived was by altarpiece commissions.
Racked on a stretcher the IV tubes string me up
Like an altarpiece I try continually to build
In order for a rapprochement with the physical body.

The Pressure

for Thomas Nash, M.D.

Too many times have I with the sun on my back, flamboyant, heinously direct,
rocked, wrung hands, my shaking head refuged in a now-wet Bounty paper towel
or institutionalized inside the free-space of my bedroom that opens like a file
on my computer screen with that which I'm constantly trying to put a name to,
the way faces in my past automatically assign to themselves signifying feelings.
Like a shot of B12 effective only if injected intramuscularly I am neutralized
as a naming vehicle by this pressure that cannot be extracted like a billboard
or wisdom tooth. No torii erects itself as gateway to the totem of experience, no
descriptive alloy exists to transform or rebirth the most primitive and bare-boned,
the referential instability of physical pain no human agency speaks successfully
in lieu of. Gritty locks felled into the sloth of tears, their salty
aftermarks imbricating my face, a kind of warrior's mask of a warrior's failure
afore the clandestine ideal of physical perfection: O poster of Marky Mark
that posits itself like an Aryan agenda against every public bus, a tableau of prayer
ossified for us to emulate. Celebrities represent what Grecian gods were once.

"Life quality" tropes the category doctors refer to with fake jocularity:
a terse smile, a quick nod, not cavalierly, really, but with no affinity either.
While I present, in crude form like an outhouse, an ideology, a practicum
my pretty breasts should make for its manifest example, but all the while
there is this pressure, iconic in nature to modify it paradoxically,
an omniscience, high-noon hot, slutty, demonic hologram embossed like Bergman's
Seventh Seal on the Silly Putty shape of my heart. The muscle adapts, adopts
the image as if the imagined face of a Bosnian orphan, the brow-swept features
twisted and bathed in a mucus for which its tiny tributary paths serve as the deaf,
dumb, and blind substitution for the mature articulation of longing and hate.
The child cries; the diastole blooms in branding exaction. The child sleeps
while pellets of sun cinder twitch and wink on the horizon; the systole
deflates, erects as if a *l'oiseau de Paradis* in order to convey
the agony of form in the rigor of its stem, or freak flowering, an ugly orange.

My physician's intelligent brow reframes behind his desk with diacritic distinction
like the beard of Zeus appearing within a cloud, a fated fetus
within the belly of its turbid future. Like a reversing falls framed and frozen,
forced to hiatus by virtue of the very process of its reversing action,
so does the pressure to live and the pressure to die halt momentarily and present,
as if a utilized gift certificate from the three wise men, a Marlboro Man genie,
the mirage-like sense of an empty room, its empirical standard; "peace of mind"

charretted into a tangible utopia, an echo–chamber of existential thought
that operates like the Mecca vision of regarding a fish tank while on morphine
where I am able to walk unbothered for a while as if along a long, white beach.
Where I am able to stand and contemplate my life, the concept and its definitions.
Where I am able to close my eyes and revel in the memory, the voice and face
the jokes, the silences, the passion, the fights, of someone I loved deeply who died.
Where trapped in the tar gut of solitary confinement I wake and am no longer blind.

I inspect my lifeline, its silly prescience, on the breathing moon–surface
of my palm, yet alert to any irregularity that might augur some imminent abortion.
The Bic fine point remains poised for further notation on the indecipherable list
of questions and comments I've arranged for this consultation, but ineffectually
for no amount of brainstorming could bulwark permanently this pressure built with
superhuman innovation and efficiency as the Egyptians did their pyramids;
before the pushing and the turning and the typhoon–like whirling starts up again.
It both buoys and sinks with me inside it, bad poem scrolled inside a Pepsi bottle,
gaining and losing, I sleep and lose sleep and rethink and rethink the perimeters,
the scientific course of which I know nothing and yet must know something by now,
more than the wet Bounty paper towel. What I know is the pressure, the stranglehold
of sadistic knees, the Devil's compression into the soles of my feet, scalding spittle
of gods that mimic my buffoonery, the bulletproof sky, the ongoing erasure of the earth
and those enfolded within it, innocuous as a tidal cove, so complacent and measured.

What I know is that the only way to stabilize is to ride through it, a raft
regaining its equilibrium in white-shark rapids, a lesser stone, bespeckled pebble
amidst a chortling brook's current or contending ego within the rock-throwing forces
dark feelings resort to in the narcissistic forum of their past belittlement.
What I know is the two rivers, the patient's and my own, that fork like a divining rod
toward some essentially healing source. What I know is that I'm both people,
one sick and one well, contending with the ongoing struggle of trying to save myself.
The x-ray glows extraterrestrial and nefarious in the late December blackness
that infiltrates my physician's office and obscures all other objects and details
other than his head, my x-ray, his desk lamp, and that strange, uncurtained window
that seems to erase all at once, in one glance, my hope of long term survival.
My torso, decapitated and cut off at the elbows, shifts in and out of focus
as if a Jane Doe resurfacing after days in the silt and oily waters of the Hudson.

"Look, an infection," my doctor declares with index finger pointed in discovery.
I blink twice, straining for recognition as I do with any picture of myself.
The shadow he refers to bursts white and translucent and upon first impression
it appeared optimistic as if a good omen were growing like an orchid in my bosom.

My impulse is to be alone with the x-ray like a loved one and the incarcerated,
to press the picture of my unhealthy lung against its double but breathing one.
What I know is the desire to resuscitate, mouth to mouth, open the dank jaws,
the partisan skin, as if beheld behind venetian blinds, zebra strips of soaked hair
and brown seaweed strewn across the face, and bring back as if to carry back in time
the fainting subject, the feminine form worn out from the fight. Her arms and feet
flag like pigeons, her weight, letter-light along my overdeveloped forearms,
their destiny as once sophomoric I dreamt it now drawn and quartered
into an array of listless limbs kicked up into a cloud, gray-blue and particle-
stained, of a hoof-clad road where a mare's distancing tail delineates
in the dusk evidence given in its disappearance, the myth of originary wholeness.

Magnetic Poetry Kit Poems

1/1/95 (8:57 pm)

Please me
and the bitter moon flooded by its shadow
repulsive but essential to the apparatus of milk
will be sweet as the winter breast of your mother's death
a sordid beauty like purple blood sprayed over a pink crushed car
a love trip then only some tiny road beneath a void momentary as rain

like whispering in a womanly weak wind
I cry without vision

2/7/95 (2:09 pm)

I ask of my blood please produce no death
though like a raw but elaborate egg you incubate in me
a woman in bed dreaming of visions so sordid
to read them would stop language as a car drives into lake water
under a rainy sky black not blue
the wind will blow after as a symphony void of music
a mother without beauty and love

how I ache in my moonless sleep
weak with madness from the storm always near
I worship waxing light, gardens, a gorgeous picture
the enormous apparatus of time from feet to head, rocks to a place above
but only bitter moans recall the urge I used to have
when beneath an essential sun never ugly or frantic
I felt what was meaningful then and must have wanted it

3/7/95 (11:45 am)

all roads drive over an enormous void like would be death
the useless picture of my head drunk & flooded underwater
as a lifetime shines above in the truly gorgeous sun
but only moonlight weak and white as breast milk do I see
falling in petals blue, pink, black, blood-rose and purple
when I stare about me into a swimming storm of winter mist then shadow

Never have I wanted from loving friends the most they can ask for
like I do today, a thousand moments crushed beneath its essential parting
from language what it must say though repulsive, delirious, raw and sordid
some hot tongue in my mad sleep may moan, whisper, scream, cry or chant

                                                        at no one

Egged on by an elaborate need to mother like a goddess the ugly within me
I manipulate out of my want the bitter gift of asking why dreams

                                                have gone away always
as if those sweet visions were still alive and easy to think of
a delicate apparatus for producing their leave-taking

                        the sadness somehow shot through with beauty
like ships who blow up atop a frantic sea recall the powerful meaning of

                                                rain and wind

5/10/95 (8:45 pm)

Black visions incubate over time in what is a bloody gorgeous head
its blue white skin motherless and drunk on thinking always about death
no gardens show their petal moment to him luscious under a forest of shadows
waxlike water here and there no sun shines delicately on the woman loved

                                                beneath
his legs, her sweet screaming stilled, gone weak and ugly
as if manipulated by someone within a tiny TV void
he licks the peach & honey breast, heaves into the sweating butt

                                chocolate smeared and easy
not the raw lust he wants but with a want only, the sad dream
                        of when he must have felt essentially powerful

bitter is beauty or love recalled it's a picture of a boy lying
                                in the road after a hit or run
never near will he be to tell of the enormous ache life has produced elaborate
                                                as fiddle music
a sordid symphony, an apparatus of urges watched but not lived from above

10/22/95 (11:40 pm)

Blue winter you and I need only to think of some moment gone but hotly here
                                                like an iron
or TV a peach rusted storm the sordid head of a madman crying out to what
                                he loves not there

18

when but for my visions used up within the fast whispering of their afterlife
would I produce heave and urge from the smelly deathwater of stopped time
them the rose the woman the friend alive & together never leave I say
                                        deliriously
to a drooling goddess repulsive though how true her shot stare do it see
be it through crushed shadows and weakest sun tongue red yet cooling her swim

I want to scream but fall behind in my blood purple bitterness I worship
                                        as if a girl's breast
not for wanting of an ugly and still raw a meaning but having felt
                                        so tiny and powerless
must take a beating beneath all the enormous lakelike lick shined sky
who drunk on play uses you next me then blows our moaning aches
                                        and delicate shadows away

7/18/97 (6:20 pm)

I ask you what essential language could manipulate into raw time
the bare void of my death   mean and elaborate as a thousand chained feet
so powerful and enormous is it   next to these tiny pink and blue moments
     only sad pictures recalled after in my head
how fast they fall like frantic petals behind me in the blood rusty road
crushed by the apparatus of shadow & bitter sky
                                        black roses incubate in their place

gifts of love   some will say   about his or hers visions of me the day
my tongue goes cool then gone   though still an urge to moan
will produce a sordid singing   a winter rain drunk   but thinking
white music   I would not read as ugly   yet no beauty can be said for
the shaking and heaving   the delicate garden bed flooded
as if by seawater   eating away the purple skin   breast and leg

there I lie but not at all within some easy acheless sleep
                                        one sweetly dreams of
no I take it on   let it stare true to life   at me from above
with a wanting   always   it never stops   the crying
                                        like a forest ripping apart
a drive I must have felt   throughout   when needs were most alive

Everybody Loves a Winner

"Freedom's just another word for nothing left to lose."
— Janis Joplin

But when you lose it's only you and the hardwood maple floor
beneath you, your shoulders pinned down, wet shirt on a clothesline
by the knees of a god leather-clad in medieval thigh-highs.
He forces you to repeat or he'll show you his fist again.
A hot pool has already boiled up in your throat —
your head to the side you watch red rivet on the polyurethane finish
the splattering on his gray T-shirt when you give him what he wants.
"Our Father who art in heaven . . ." and you've got to get it right,
no tone of sacrilege, nothing but the pure submission
that the purgatorial twilight outside has brought about,
this epic plot eschatological in proportion
where you are the dot in a pointillist painting,
the undetectable one, the point of vanishing.
The streaks of amethyst and taupe underscore the sky's authenticity.
It's hard to believe that you ever thought it beautiful.
Hasn't reality always been by virtue of the realistic aspect always horrible
like the real rope that ties your ankles and wrists together,
prepared like the modern-day equivalent of a virgin for slaughter,
a stiff strapped to a cake of cement en route to the East River
and you can't feel anything from your pelvis on down;
you look forward to nothing in totality now that your options have run out.

Everybody loves a winner, but when you lose it's just you and the partial view
out the hospital window, just you in front of the doctor when he tells you
you're too hopeful, just you and less than that for you're shrinking, melting,
you are that which is diminishing like a snow bank in February
like the wicked witch of the west destroyed by drinking water,
just you and the self-conscious stratum of your prayers
where, in its tapestry, you are less than water and the verdigris thread
that depicts the facial details of those who will go on without you
the winners with torsos built with such genetic supremacy
they appear manufactured, checked once for efficiency like an Icelandic horse
then set free like wild ponies on the Cote d'Azur.
Everybody loves a winner but when you lose it's you who's watching the ponies,
your individuality instantly annihilated in the category of spectatorship,
drowning in the oceanic still life that backdrops their wildness,

the waves pitched in churlish peaks like cake frosting or moussed hair,
the trends of teal and navy like the subway map of your body's meridians
for all of life has becomes paradigmatic of your interiority in its finitude,
the seminary belfry the diagrammatic sonata for the intricacy of your despair
this particular December evening when you actually feel the winners gather
together in the chapel and an hour later in the mess hall
and mutter their gratitude for genetic technology and the more secure
sense of community it's produced like electric fencing.
When you lose it's just you watching the electric fence, like a cow
with your flat brow and slightly furrowed brown eyes that steady themselves
as only a sign from which no signification can be wrought
not by theologian, semiotician, vegetarian, or third-generation farmer.
Oblivious to the slaughter number tattooed on their ears as their
nostrils flare in the just-above-freezing air, they watch the humans
scurry back to the hutch where a singular trail of chimney smoke promotes
a sense of gradation and process amidst a darkness that descends
in one monolithic and monochromatic movement like the guillotine.

Everybody loves a winner, but when you lose it's just you and your bedroom
as an antechamber, the snuffbox of the bed itself where like ash inside
a mastaba you have already returned to white powder. I have returned already
to Mecca, to Minnesota, to my future fast-forwarded in the multiminute
of my being forced to focus on my mortality at such a young age
like the repeated refrain of a psychopathic rapist to keep him from raping me
I'll stare into the pupil, the dilating finality, a kind of metaphysical duel
where the stakes pierce themselves like harpoons into what's purely physical
and win by deferral, by a Buddhist acknowledgment of the world's inequality
and return already, ahead of schedule, to fray from fabric, to tree from text.
I'll watch the wild ponies from an aisle seat in business class
that flies solo sans 747 chassis, having already experienced the crash.
I'll win by losing, by looking up at the winning sky from a six-sided box
for nothing is lonelier than a grave, mass or single, shallow or deep
determined or ubiquitous like the eccentric wish for the at-last
unfettered ashes to be sprinkled like fairy dust over a favorite mountain range.
I'll give birth to myself by virtue of my degradation,
lick the self-inflicted wounds of my masochism,
carry a pea on my nose in the effort to perfect my posture
and take it on the chin as the British would say.
I'll lose by winning, take the sky like a phallus into my mouth
and subsume what's impossible to subsume by the degree of my subordination.
Everybody loves a winner, loves the credit card, gold or green,

when it's taken out to pay for dinner.   Everybody loves the New Jersey upstart,
the unmanicured beauty, the wizened scholar who's revered in part
for his hideous appearance.   And everybody loves Magic Johnson
even more than ever now that he's HIV positive.
But they don't love my dead friends, and they don't love me either.
They don't love a loser unless you were first good at athletics.
Everybody loves a winner.   I love them true myself.
It's just that I recognize the loser from my own lonesome state,
one tree to another, from across a forest, the matte green tennis lawn
at Wimbledon, like "Some Enchanted Evening", as having won at something else.

Omen

for Sharon Olds

White roses winter into human depth —
into shit with us, their dry petals and tireless leaves.

They return in fleets as if to nascence.
Migrating, they spur an infinite helix, like a snail's shell or DNA.

Yet into a position so wretched and twisted
their rigor mortis appears, at the same time, unnatural.

Blankly they stare, panicked, spotlighting the indoor air,
perpetually in recognition of that, their assassin:

White into black into white into black into white into no more.
Only desperate scratches are left to decipher on the floor.

I've been trying to trust since I was an atom.
Indeed, the very explosion of cells in me serves as an example.

Doesn't my sleeping spine submit to recontouring on the Seaman mattress?
And offered up half-shelled and therefore raw in expression

My sustained scatological admiration for the death of white roses
provides another just as loathsome and handsome.

Make Costly Your Tears

The great ceiling spreads before me, wings of a pterodactyl,
blank as our concept of heaven and as absolving,
with its absorbent powers.

Droplets of Steuben flow upward from my eyes,
lend a semi-gloss sheen to my perception.
I almost prefer the world this way, encased in my sorrow
since that is the manner in which I keep you invincible.

This is only morning. The sink bowls before me, a porcelain cavern.
Do I regret the profuse knowledge I've gained of your body?
How well clothes hide us! There's never a need to feel self-conscious.

We no longer live in the age of letters.
If we did I would have yours tied up somewhere
for the purpose of experiencing a surge of pure eroticism
(usually made opaque from my affections)
when rewitnessing their confinement.

As a culture, cursively, we've denominated into signatures.
Yours, in blue Magic Marker, stenciled throughout my field of vision.
I'm able to stare for a remarkably long time at your signed name,
practicing the art of minimalism,
as if the letters could give way at last, like my legs did, like a dam,
to their signification,
though I love the sign anyway, even without its meaning:
your cock was made for my mouth.

Steuben stands the hardest to break of all glass.
I've collected my tears in a pan like gravel.
May they pave driveways with utilitarian humility someday,
learning effacement by virtue of their production.
May they give way to tread marks like legs or signatures,
leave a stark mark of erasure on the honorary Firestone.

Now I understand how I got into this rattrap of wistfulness.
Nothing sets us up more for disappointment than twilight.
From the start we are predisposed to idealization by reality,
by its exquisite and erratic and incompassionate nature.

Family Romance

for Adrienne Rich

Whenever I catch two men kiss, in the streets, or in the movies,
I'm filled with so much envy, always wanting to be filled up
the way a woman would. Their jaws interlock as if to kill —
true, it was a lioness that I saw suffocate a wildebeest once —
but the depths of their tongues that churn round in the caves
of their mouths like fornicating hips or shamans writhing with prayer
before the primordial campfire, I recognize parasitically
for I can only feminize, exiled to the inversion of this passion.
If hell is starvation, then always from me the carrot of equanimity
gleams in its linear superiority, born on my knees, as it were.
I serve in abstention, help throw into high relief like Mt. Rushmore
"the great" through representation of "the mediocre", of the mother,
of earthen conjugation freshly seeded whether or not barren I remain.

Although, I too know the friction of torso against my skin,
rubbed against the pecs of my breasts, flexed tendons like a horse's neck.
I've lubricated my fist up to my elbow with the best of them;
and suckled a man's tits as roughly as if he were a woman and I a lesbian.
I've witnessed his eyes roll back into his head with breathy subjugation.
But I am, alas, like their enemy, their opposite, yet not their equal
fraught from the fission of the first human into something quite different
preamble to their totem the way canine compares to Neanderthal,
(albeit constructed just as much from advertising as from genetics).
The desire I elicit expedites, perhaps, more the social than the libidinal,
more the shelter than the landscape, more the exodus than the Zionist sky.

More the wingnut in the economical structure of the nuclear unit
than the shark blue heat of locomotion that's black in feeling,
the *double entendre* that's entropy and beauty: an x-ray of an elderly hand
stacked upon an x-ray of my young heart blueprints my future, shark blue.
To kiss that hand with love in my heart is what I'll spend a lifetime doing;
to swallow my innocence whole in the process like a goldfish,
to respect the fraternity, to respect the beating.
But I can never sleep with my father throughout history and make history,
even though my father fucks me, perfunctorily,
the inferior prerequisite to actualized oratory, the smoking of his cigar.
Absorbed by history as nonpartisan, as audience by auditorium,
as ingredient by compound, as the wildcard, postmodern elaboration of a rib,

piecemealed to more skeletal paraphernalia in the Natural Museum

I'm never the museum, nor the tautological exhibit, nor the curatorial whim.

I'm the freak of each, hybrid of anything, the Epiphany of orgasmic peaking,

the dog in the snuff film shot in real time by bastardized time.

I'm the moon when there's no moon forced to regard the world's lack of night.

I'm the dismembered arm in a Jasper Johns, pre-Raphaelite

without predisposition myself, a perigee forever without point of contact.

Like the lake that reflects the sky as it pathologically lies about God,

I'm more than water and reflection and rest amidst churlishness for the eye.

I'm more than a wingnut, than open arms or open legs or a bottomless throat.

I'm more than the man who mounts deep inside the man, inside me, the woman.

I'm both the truth and the lie about God.

I'm both but I'm not a hermaphrodite, nor a cross-dresser, nor do I lip-sync

"Stormy Weather" at the Hellfire Club on Ladies Night.

I'm both the id like the lake, mum and blind,

and the hyperbolic superego of the sky, tyrannically weak.

I'm both the night and a particle of the night, animadverted into annihilation.

I'm both the shark and the x-ray, my future and the elderly hand.

I'm both the killer and the lover, the father and the lioness.

I'm both the Acropolis and the gorgeous disengagement of the Parthenon.

Palea

Only my mouth taking you in, the greenery splayed deep green.

Within my mouth, your arm inserted, a stem of gestures, breaking gracefully.

Into each other we root arbitrarily, like bushes, silken and guttural.

Palaver, we open for the thrill of closing, for the thrill of it: opening.

The night was so humid when I knelt on the steps, wet and cold, of prewar stone.

A charm bracelet of sorts we budded, handmade but brazen, as if organic.

I cannot imagine the end of my fascination, emblazoned but feather-white too.

The gold closure of this like a gold coin is, of course, ancient.

Why can't experience disseminate itself, be silken and brazen yet underwater?

A miniature Eiffel Tower, an enameled shamrock, a charm owned by its bracelet.

The Crying Game

written to the song by Geoff Stevens

in memory of my father

I know all there is to know about the crying game

    for I've seen him turn   his face
away from me

So now I can say I've seen the lord,
                              his aquiline nose
his long sandy blond hair streaked with blue and red
No tears were streaming   down *his* cheeks

    When he turned his back to me
    the great V of his torso pivoted   like the turning point in a
                                        classical novel
as Anna foresaw the train tracks   in Frou Frou's broken back

I've discovered my eventual absence in his sacrum
the thick braid of muscle that   denotes into nothing

I've had my share   of the crying game

    when I watched his body turn, slowly
as a rotation of the earth
                         or screw in a head press
first there are kisses
then there are sighs

his effeminate waist   swiveled in its socket
            of the pelvis that once fit me   like a yoke

his body covering me, a critical mass
the pressure of his hand,   before my confirmation
           barely felt the way a priest blesses a child

  pushing me down, further and further

to my confirmation, the denigration of a child
as if swallowing the semen of god would bring me closer to gods

and then before you know where you are
                              you're saying goodbye

O they say he loves us all   but for some reason   he stopped loving me

One day soon I'm going to tell the moon   about the crying game
and we'll cry together   like the day I told my father   I was HIV positive

And if he knows maybe he'll explain
                              just him and me   under a fluorescent tube
our chairs as close as we could push them together

            why there are heartaches
            why there are tears

If I had been younger he would have embraced me   with his whole body
held me in his lap while I sobbed and he,
                though less dramatically, too

            He'll know what to do
            to stop feeling blue

but the closest we could come to   that was to cry together   but separately

      our heads in our individual hands, though our knees remained touching
for crying is always,   in essence, about crying alone

                  when love disappears

into the astringent light of fluorescence

first there are kisses, then there are sighs
then fluorescent light replaces the moon

            I genuflect   beneath the circular tube
      lit 24 hours, a postmodern shrine
                        that illuminates my deathbed
            spare and   apologetic

                        bare futon on a wood floor
I'm willing to be yoked by his pelvis again instead of,   instead of . . .

but he doesn't look back, he doesn't   say why
Then before you know where you are

                              you're saying goodbye

Don't want no more
     of the purifying, of the placating, of the penury ritual
of self-deprivation of the crying game, the goals, overly ambitious,
of its refinement like spiritual fasting for which fasting, broth and
bread, then bread and water, then just water, only water, itself will
not provide a spiritual dimension, an exaltation that results from
impoverishment, base in expectation, ingenuous in intent by being void
of intent, of sacrificial ecstasy comprised of only one desire, only one
like water, a fasting of desires until living upon one, desiring only one
desire, the desire for atonement is only that

Don't want no more
     of the nights, not just the sweats, not just the fear of sweats,
not just the dreams, the gargantuan, exhaustive dreams, the hallways,
the staircases, the crowds, the water, the betrayal, not just their
cruel non sequiturs of composition, not just the bedside light turned on
at four in the morning as if of its own accord, contemptuously, in order
to underscore the aloneness, "You must feel so alone," it says, without
affection, without even a gesture, "You must feel so alone," it says
mechanically undergoing modes of observation like a night nurse
blanched to the moans of her patients. She reads my unconscious fears as if
viewing an x-ray of them, a blood pressure speedometer, then checks them
off, executing the little marks on her chart with cursory but automatic
precision simultaneously shutting off another light with each notation.
It's the crying game when she's left, it's the squeaks of her rubber-soled
white shoes on the linoleum as she whisks onward down the corridor into
silence. It's the length of darkness ahead I'm forced to contemplate. It's
the drive for relief that refuses to atrophy

Don't want no more
     of the condoms, of policing, of elaborating excuses, of newsbreaking,
of the crying game that bullies me into one crying jag after another with
no reprieve to be found after, of vitamins, of poems, of suicidal scenarios,
of imagining, willing your life to change but nothing happens, no parole,

no tenure, no wedding, just a waiting, the massive silence of a crowd waiting
the silence of exodus, the silence of entrapment, the silence of failed
imaginings: hungry mouths in an orphanage

Don't want no more
    of what I can't have no more of, of the paradigm of the crying game
which is the paradigm of starvation driven so deep inside me it's written
infinitely in the mutilation of my body, separating me, irreparably from
myself, so left I am to keep vigil over a kind of vegetable, a love death,
a death wish that can't fulfill itself, that just keeps hanging on like
Karen Ann Quinlan

Clash

As if without agony the white convertible, a Mustang, peels along,
pierces the chiffon-thin dawn, sheet by sheet,
white as white chocolate or a snow leopard's spots.

Far off people make love and moan as if in great pain,
but they're not, though their pleasure be pitched at an undetectable level
like a whistle only dogs can hear.

And I, as if a dog, hear it all,
hued yet whole in its spectrum, a hologram Xeroxed to perfection
where the exaction of exhaust exhalation and heaves of passion
stack this cruel world upon its cruelty.
Their secretions smear their loins like white chocolate,
and from their eyes spurt white tears of pity.

I both watch and want to stop
the lovemaking bodies that wriggle with self-centered abandon
deep inside my body the way a dream does or hope will despite my cynicism;
pulling me to move by collar and chain
within my emotionlessness, motionless as a parked car,
a white convertible, a snow leopard devoured by dogs,
I both watch and want to stop.

What Calendars Have Become

When you're sick the months merge, first the seasons, then the years
the movement of time transforming into the plaything of others,
which voyeuristically you witness as if at leisure for such pastimes.
You regard with faltering bemusement the numerical delineation of days
and weeks as they organize themselves so aggressively on some boring
Sierra Club Calendar . . . the one that hangs in the blood lab, for instance —

You stare with morbid blankness at time demystified by such practical
factors — its perfect arc appears less grand and therefore hopeful,
aware now that it's your body only that's the means of measuring the future —
Hence all else becomes superfluous and surreal: goals, dreams, desires —
strange accoutrements, mostly media-induced, of our particular culture.

With effort you recall the ambition you once matched in its swift exiting
of days marked with giants X's or efficient little checks — when time continually
reconfigured itself before your eyes like yoga masters demonstrating
the many venues of Kundalini orgasm. Looking at a calendar now is like
turning the large, brightly colored pages of some coffee table accessory —

the intensity of pattern in the shrine-like boudoirs hurts your eyes
for a moment as sudden daylight does for those resistant to reality.
You strain to adjust, then regret the small feat of assimilation —
your regard registers as dull compared to their fascinating accomplishments of
coordination and wild self-involvement. Perhaps your index fingers traces
a stray hand back to the shoulder, the magical displacement of limbs leading
to anxiety and confusion — and a jealousy unlike anything previously experienced.

Jealous of what, exactly? The multiple thrill, the unmannered mastery,
the treasure map of the many pleasure points and unerring, navigational ability?
The barrier of skin and how it used to signify sex, an eroticism triggered in merely
the anticipation of boundary-crossing? — When ill, perimeters of privacy close down
methodically — intrusion therapy having been taken to its extreme — like veins, for
instance. Initially technicians were glad to see me, until my veins began to
systemically collapse — and I became difficult to "access", the value
of my interiority a summation of only that: blood rivers to be tapped —
nobody wants to keep seeing someone's face in this kind of circumstance.

Examining the lovers, it's hard to believe that such control over pleasure exists —
when the organic production of pain from disease progression flourishes gratuitously,

the way wildflowers engendered by bone grist and bile might connect us to a larger
schematic and with it a sense of cohesiveness — a lack of ultimate futility — but the
wildflower, say the edelweiss blossom, in its figurative smallness and isolation,
cannot act as the horizon does or vanishing point in a painting by piecing
together such grandiose abstraction. It remains small and isolated in our one-on-one
viewing, a kind of consultation that eventually flatlines, like the strategy sessions
with my doctor — his white coat, the edelweiss, my body, the testing ground of science.

Whatever the essential self once was disappears before you slowly over time
before the polite and caring physician, before the scale, the ridiculing mirror
as the body is given over, slowly, like the minds of the brainwashed to covert
operations or information from the interrogated when given sufficient amount of
torture — like the broken will of a rape victim; veterans of war to symbolic cloth.
To medical intervention — drugs, procedures — I have bequeathed myself.

This is the kind of agenda that calendars have become, grids that pretend to connect
but actually disassociate us from the problematic of essential meaning. Sadly their
arbitrary thematics, i.e., Jackson Pollock paintings, famous writers at their desks,
dreary watercolors so mediocre they're unable to distinguish winter from summer — twelve
months, four seasons, 365 days, 24 hours, merely provide a means of distraction from
the feelings of senselessness and disorientation, the whys of fluke beginnings and ends
of existence, the concept of an overarching trajectory to guide us, to comfort and
to protect our idea of importance — the intrinsic value of mankind as contextualized by
human history — disguising, as necrophilia does lifelessness, our aeonian worthlessness.

It's as if one were perpetually forced to witness the crashing of a plane,
to view the cruel and surreal sequencing that occurs within the depressurized cabin.
And by virtue of this raw and honest demonstration, any pretense of enlightenment
reveals in the end — as white sheet does a corpse, as corpse does the anatomy
specimen, as anatomy specimen, the banal fatuousness of an overdetermined soul — the
falsehood of comprehension; for whatever is spontaneously or in turn assiduously
understood instantaneously dismantles, suctioned back into that fractured space, the
black hole from which it originated: passengers and passenger paraphernalia alike
equalized by disaster when the airborne exit door unexpectedly lurches open and into
the ravenous vacuum, purses, raincoats, briefcases, high-heeled shoes ricochet
like billiards against metal armrests and the heavy plastic of upper compartments
before bursting in fits and spirals unto the white, even-tempered glare of oblivion.

Our dead faces are born already inside us. They float just beneath the surface of our
expressions, joyful and despairing, like lily pads asphyxiated in a frozen pond.
Some fail quickly while some fail incrementally with time to absorb

all the infinitesimal disappointments, the details, gory and beautiful, reflected
in the shocked face continually reframed by the realization of its death forthcoming.
Its features document the difference between a fatal accident and wasting away . . . the
excruciatingly slow entry into the self-dug abyss like Eskimo elders excommunicated from
the community — their footprints filling up immediately with fresh snow — evidence
that the heavens are in agreement, acknowledged now and then in empty-canteen silence.
Glancing over his shoulder, perhaps one contemplates the humility of return, the
slaughter by his family for carnal nourishment — there is no sparing. But all suffering
mitigates in severity when compared to this loneliness, all suffering preferable
to the withholding quiescence of snow falling, exponentially, upon fallen snow.

I'm surprised to know that it's beautiful where I'm headed. The black-and-white
photographs do not do it justice. Dogs barking in the distance urge me toward it.
I hear them continuously, regardless of their actual presence, noise itself eventually
representing them, both bus breaks and sparrows. There is no design behind it,
no skeletal structure that spits ultraviolet fire beneath ambitious footsteps
like some other kind of subway system; no elaborate tapestry to which we should remain
gratefully stupefied aside from this tapestry of landscape and its magnetic fourth
dimension pulling us toward it like passengers and their paraphernalia out of a
depressurized cabin — an underground undifferentiated from the ambiguity of clouds
and cloudless light and darkness sometimes punctuated by stars and sometimes pitch.

I keep forgetting it's not a personal defeat to be so sick.
What was once a mind for music and words has become an amateur mad-scientist,
an expert at needle gauging — butterfly 25 if you're going for the hand —
an evolutionary step up from rat or chimp for drug protocols called obnoxiously
"cocktails" by the reading public (a joke on gays, I'm certain) — I honor the demands
of earthbound stasis that pulsates with monotone enthusiasm as if an artificially
resuscitated patient whose pupils rooted and dilated persist in their brain-dead state
to stare with dumb depth at the futureless sky of the hospital ceiling
and its inability to defend and therefore redeem the world — regardless of the
Styrofoam squares either stained or missing, or the fluorescent tube twitching
on and off its illumination overhead or further down the corridor —

I refer to the world but I speak of the body. I want my body to reassure me,
my catheterized limbs to start signing madly in the air, swallows flapping
to free themselves. Teach me, *Sensei* — my body — , teach me,
with *sang-froid* impartiality as you have all my life about the meaning of life,
teach me as you did once of athletic executions, the thrill of unskilled kicking
in lake water, teach me as you did of sexual collusion, the pure suspense
of someone touching, that way, my skin, painful and exciting like running into a

forest at midnight, my hair caught in branches, withered leaves abusing my face.
(I ran faster, willfully, into its dimensions darkening as if blindfolded — of course.)

You were always much braver than I, my body, as if mounted upon you but reinless
I were. You reared, your sinewy legs, your baleful eyes, your wildlife mane,
long striding away from the barn, breath crystallizing in the cold from soft nostrils.
The challenge to stay alive was the challenge to trust you — not as simple
as it sounds — and it was a sound, not singular or melodic, not a narrative or refrain,
not a language, nothing to be translated or negotiated, but a voice nonetheless
unimaginable, imperceptible, absolute, archetypal, to which I had to listen carefully
as carefully as I must listen to it now, left ear to the earth for approaching hooves.
It's us returning, more in love than ever, near collapse in the somatic blackout that
signifies death. It's us. Moonlight beats down upon the barn as if it were a crèche.

Teach me now about time running out — about clocks and calendars, and hourglasses,
and sundials, mechanisms for measuring the chasm, the adorable, the heinous duration,
leading up to this process of time running out. I have come to the part where I must
overcome my failing — teach me, *Sensei*, how to leave, how to say goodbye to you.
Help push into the river the handmade canoe of birchbark we rocked together,
like a *Todtenbaum*, its ebb as effortless as levitation, me from you or vice versa.
See me through this juncture to the threshold waiting like a waterfall ahead,
Flesh I have loved like no other. Don't let it hurt. Don't let it be too quiet.

Teach me, one foot in front of the other, this last mortal action, basic, necessary
the way you once did to chew bread or drink water, O body of reason.
Assume again with me a dead man's float or corpse position in yoga.
Relax my limbs, salve my anxiety: talk back to me like the friend you've been.

My mind draws a blank. My heart beats mundanely. I'm supposed to be glad and accepting
but I'm at a loss for last lines, final sentences of closure that would convince me —
of what, I don't know. It's not as if I ask for some proof of an afterlife
or some strange and worthy purpose upon which at one time I insisted, against
my better judgment and intuition, must concur with physical suffering —
some apex achieved in terms of moral purification, humility, and patience.

Take my left hand into my right — and soothe me, *Sensei*, release me from the need
for something delicate and original — and sincere enough (like chance, or love, or
peace, or humanity) — to make this worth it. Only the knowing of you could be that.
This leaving that is your liberation, please make it mine also.

RIP, My Love

Let us be apart then like the panoptical chambers in ICU
patient X and patient Y, our names Magic Markered hurriedly on cardboard
and taped pell-mell to the sliding glass doors, "Mary", "Donald", "Tory";
an indication that our presence there would prove beyond temporary, like snow flurry.
Our health might be regained if aggressive medical action were taken, or despite
these best efforts, lost like missing children in the brambles of poor fortune.
The suffering of another I can only envision through the mimesis of my own,
the alarming monitor next door in lieu of a heartbeat signifying cardiac arrest,
prompts a scurry of interns and nurses, their urgent footsteps to which
I listen, inert and prostrate, as if subject to the ground tremors of
a herd of buffalo or horses, just a blur in the parched and postnuclear distance.
I listen, perhaps the way the wounded will listen to the continuing war,
so different sounding than before, the assault of noise now deflected against
consciousness rather than serving as motivation for patriotism and targets.
Like fistfuls of dirt loaded with pebbles and rocks thrown at my front door,
I knew that the footsteps would soon be running to me also.
The blood pressure cuff swaddled around my arm pumped in its diastolic state
independently like an iced organ ready for transplant
as I witnessed with one circular rove of my eyes my body now dissected
into television sets, like one of those asymmetrical structures
that serves as a model for a molecular unity in elementary science classes.
And the plastic bags of IV fluids that hung above me, a Miro-like mobile or iconic toy
for an infant's amusement, measured the passing of time by virtue of their depletion.
Sometimes I could count almost five and then seven swinging vaguely above me at 4 a.m.
I remember the first, hand-held high above me when I arrived via ambulance at the ER, the
gurney accelerating as a voice exclaims on the color of my hands, "They're *blue!*"
Another voice (deeper) virtually yells out into the chaos that she can't get a pulse.
Several pairs of scissors begin simultaneously to cut off my clothes, their shears
working their way upward like army ants from pant cuff and shirtsleeve,
a formulaic move for the ER staff which, despite its routine, still retains
a sense of impromptu in the hurriedness of the cutting both deft and crude,
in the sound of their increased breathing, of their efforts intensified by my blood
pressure dropping, the numbers shouted out as if into night fog and ocean.
It's not a lack of professionalism but the wager of emotional investment that I feel.
One attendant, losing her aplomb for a moment, can't contain herself from remarking
(as if I'm already post-mortem) on what a great bra I have;
"Stretch lace demi-cup, Victoria's Secret," I respond politely in my head.
In turn, when they put the oxygen tube into my nose I thought immediately
of Ali McGraw on her deathbed in *Love Story* and how good she looked in one.

And then the catheter where I pissed continually into a bottle like a paraplegic
let me in on the male fear of castration,
my focus centered entirely on that tube, its vulnerable rigging
which I held onto tenderly throughout the night like something dying
against my thigh or something birthing. I held on though the IV in my forearm
overextended with a kind of pleading, the needle hooked deep into a mainstream vein
the way in deep-sea fishing lines are cast into the darkest water,
my body thrashing about in the riverweed of its fluids.
The translucent infrastructure of IVs and oxygen tubes superimposed itself upon me
like a body double, more virulent and cold, like Leda pinned and broken by her swan,
like the abandoned and organ-failed regarding its superior soul ascend.
So completely and successfully reconfigured within its technological construct
my body proper no longer existed, my vital signs highlighted in neon
preceded the spiraling vortex of my interiority,
the part of me people will say later that that's what they loved
when they roam about in the cramped rare book library of their memory
for a couple of minutes and think of "Tory".
Movement can be accounted only in shadows, Virilio informs us,
the reconciliation of oneself in one's disappearance.
An anachronistic sundial, I turn my profile
and the fluorescence falls unfractured, unmediated onto the postmodern tenebrism
of absence against absence, my quickened inhalations against my backless gown.
My love for you, my love, for my friends, untethers and floats,
snaps apart and off me like the IV tubes and monitor wires
the flailed arms of an octopus unfolding without gravity,
as I reach up in a Frankensteinian effort to shut off my monitors,
the constant alarming of the human prototype my own body keeps rejecting,
while death moves closer, a benign presence.
It stands respectfully just outside the perimeters of my life
and adjusts itself the way the supervising nurse did the monitor perimeters
to suit my declining vital signs so I could get some sleep.
I felt a relationship with death, a communication, it was more familiar
than I ever imagined, what I had always returned to as the sign of me, the self
we attribute to the mysterious and perfectly ordered Romantic notion of origin.
What I'm trying to say is that it was not foreign. It was not foreign,
but it was not a homecoming either.
There was no god, no other land, no beyond;
no amber, no amethyst, no avatar.
But there was a suspension, there was an adieu to recognition
to the shoes of those I love, like Van Gogh's, a pair but alone
the voices of loved ones, their tones, their intonations, like circulation,

close–circuited but effective.

There was a listless but clear–thinking comfort that into my own eyes

I would go, although not "into" in the Bachelardian sense

which implies diminishment; there was none of that.

It was just the opposite: expansion but without a pioneer's vision.

What we regard as the "self" extended itself, but I wouldn't say in a winged way,

over the Bosch–like landscape of brutal interactions

and physical pain and car alarms and the eternal drilling of disappointment

the exigent descendence of everyday that every day you peer down or up

its daunting staircase, nauseous with vertigo

gathering like straw the rudimentary characteristics of courage, gumption, innovation

and faking it to the hilt like a hilarious onslaught of sham orgasms.

Transcendence might be the term Emerson would lend it.

What I'm trying to say is that it wasn't lonely.

II.

Cinéma Vérité

Cinéma Vérité

Like great moments in filmmaking when Brando adheres his wad
of ACG (already chewed gum) under the iron balcony and parodies
the decline of late twentieth-century Europe with this gesture.

Or the closing scene in *Contempt* where the minuscule Fiat
white as Bardot's bleach job collides fatalistically and thus hubristically
with a trailer truck and her neck, white as a Fiat, snaps
at once instantaneous and infinite like the bereavement sobs of Juno
at four in the morning that register as silent to sleeping mortals.

You within the context of your death must diminish in value like the ruble
within a capitalist market, a fag smoldering, chartreuse and laconic
within solitary confinement, despite my enshrining efforts to embalm you
which assert themselves as indecipherable as asphalt amidst asphalt.

The way in Warhol's *Empire*, shot (almost) in real time,
diminishment occurs by virtue of real time as if the incarcerated spectator
were forced to keep vigil over the last eight hours of the Empire State
Building's life — a kind of iconic sublimation into abstraction takes place,
where the cheap film posits, projects a silkscreen, a replicate, an aberration
and the Empire becomes a sign for itself, for the signified of abstraction,
of abyss, a negative that foregrounds its positive like the Venus de Milo,
a stationary torso suspended like the skull as locus in Hamlet's soliloquy,
the moon as telos for our displacement from the last reel of utter darkness.
The Empire, glistening as if the teeth of the dead, rises, exhumed
like Houdini or Jesus or Elizabeth Barrett Browning
from a neuter desert, the impossible tomb
of its representation, and incinerates in homage to itself
like the actual cremation of your body.

According to a sadist's definition of "slowly"
as in torture, as in interrogation, where the voice of confession
becomes the belated product, a fetish accoutrement, of its oppressor
the libido frees itself like a holocaust survivor
and the world, poor and empty as the final frame in *The Passenger*
where the clay terrain, the barking dog, the shrunken sky
become merely the fetishistic accoutrements of poverty and emptiness.
I see my future through the eyes of that Jack Nicholson.

O in Oshima's *In the Realm of the Senses* when Sada castrates Kichi
after his death, I want to keep you like that, your cock preserved
like the brain of a genius, beyond bronze, pickled in a jar of formaldehyde.
"That movie's about castration," you said.
"That movie's about possession," I said. It's about both, together and cut
(the word "togetherness" a pun on "alone" and "cut" in Japanese).
During a course of phone calls I tracked down your body like a death sheriff
on its post-mortem itinerary from mortician to medical examiner to crematorium
in an effort to discover your final resting place, much the way Dustin Hoffman
à la *The Graduate* pathfinds the church where Elaine is getting married
but minus the macabre intent of this necrophiliac's obsession.
What I would have given: blank check, right hand, first book of poetry,
to intervene, to interrupt, to slip surreptitiously into the funeral home,
nauseous from the redolence of absenteeism, and lick intrepidly
without a time limit, the irregularly sewn sutures from the autopsy incisions.
Your handsome head albeit turbid in recognition remains stationary, the bust
of Mahler by Rodin, the bleeding feet of Christ in their oracular hemorrhage.
If granted the opportunity I would have asked, I would have pleaded
as the prime minister's wife did with the wife of Saddam Hussein
who received the next day in lieu of his life, the body parts of her husband
parceled in three Hefty lawn bags.

Today is the anniversary of when we last saw each other. Turning the corner
your face lit up like Northumberland terrain idealized by a Northumbrian.
But the earth and its oral traditions serve now only to disappoint me
as do my friends, as does UPS, as does the road, winding or freeway,
in light of the Jacobean erasure of that expression; the snapshot I'll not have.
We stood where the clouds colluded in a tenet of unsurpassed fatalism
flattering to our star-crossed desires as the dream of duet suicide.
We experienced our corporeality fail us then, conversely, in the pleasure
of touching, for we are not, like sanitized forceps, touching now.
We are not, like forsythia and lake water, touching now.
Corporeality failed us both even though only one of us died.
Corporeality, at once omniscient and estranged, deauthenticates the body
in its urgency to prove itself otherwise the way newscasting does world events
the way a cemetery betrays the closure of death with touchstones for eternity.
Corporeality humiliates us as if expelled from flesh afore flesh we're forced
as a dog is to defecate in public, to watch interminably our expulsion
until pathetic I admit congeals the bodily composition that cannot bring you back,
my hand, a peg in its ineffectualness to make real this lowly a handmade wish.

Once when I called you after the fact (it's sick, I know) just to hear you "live"
like a cassette of Maria Callas' unknown recordings I own, it worked, so to speak,
your outgoing message, regardless of the emptiness, both pythogenic and Arcadian
the way one engages in part in phone sex to reacquaint the self with its extremes,
a tautological erotica, where the moment more than emblematizes the history,
but is its emblem as if to withhold it, bury it in an arcanum like your remains
the body I never got to identify that, now cremated, endures as unidentifiable;
a kind of déclassé epiphany. And I wonder if the void, the arcanum, itself
provides perversely the means for its so-called fulfillment like an artifact,
like a fetish accoutrement, like an icon, like a national flag, like a Wonderbra,
like a lock of your hair where a kind of double death occurs upon discovery,
the way masturbating to the memory of a dead man becomes the only way to climax.

When I called a few days later, your telephone had been temporarily disconnected
and I flew in reaction throughout the corridors of my refractive identity
like Julie Christie in *Darling* who throws a shit fit in the Italian villa
when she finds it impossible to reach the insipid Count, her husband
hyperventilating from the sheer existential pitch of her isolation:
her poor choice in marriage, her inevitable aging, her preposterous décolletage.
I breathe in deeply the sickly air of a city plagued by an august siesta.
Your death augurs a boundlessness, isotropic as saline.
I mourn you, suspended like Sappho, from the balcony of my future,
iced out amidst the vulgar silence, cruel and penetratingly so by definition.
The balcony, a baroque catastrophe (not unlike the one Brando sullies
before he dies in *Last Tango in Paris*) protrudes as if a stillborn pregnancy
over a centennial nothing, an ocean debased in celluloid.

One day I'll make a little pilgrimage to your burial site.
I'll travel incognito, via a Greyhound, sporting Jackie O. sunglasses
and a platinum flip-do wig, exercising thus the bad faith intrinsic to selfhood
in a flagrant display of its inherent exhibitionism.
Therefore most true to the emotive content which propelled this journey I'll be,
closest to the person whom you loved when I peer myopically to inspect your name.
It makes no sense to me, staring a bit longer, just a mirage of letters engraved
that contain the secret of your name like an anagram or dream condensation.
I work hard to interpret, regardless of the snow and unusually high wind
still searching like a mammal for a carcass I've witnessed thrown to the wolves
yet I can't get over a land like this that refuses to hand you, its hostage, back.
I hate the complacent woods, the recalcitrant answering machine,
the patronizing sky that pretends to understand while denying you ever existed.
I picture you in Canada, proud to have staged so successfully your death,

(and in a way you did, for as children of Watergate we know what to erase)
where behind your computer screen you're in command again
with a newfangled modem which not only promises a modicum of control
over earthly events way back when virtual reality merely assimilated,
but allows voyeuristic predilections to be transferentially indulged ad infinitum.
You type in your name and it takes you to your grave. You recognize instantly
the pitiful sight of the sentimentally driven woman in the wig.
You watch the larger than life tears like Man Ray's famous photograph
freeze-frame in their initial debouchment then rivet through the granite crevices
of your birth and death dates, obscured by mascara, blue-tinted.
You feel love, then fear, guilt, anger, then helplessness. Your anxiety peaks
but you resist temptation to stroke F7 and eliminate the image.
Then you think of something to say, something both protective and productive
like "Tory, when was the last time you backed up your files?"
The woman reflexes either from a sudden sense of cold or dissident sound
but not from this lame attempt you figure, articulating the self-recrimination
"lame attempt" out loud. She returns to reverie while you watch her like wildlife.
The modem provides then the cache of an unexpected benefit
and you're able to read, like subtitles, verbatim the thoughts in her brain.
Intrigued by a breach in the epistolary canon this method of discourse may provoke
not to depreciate the motivation to speak, the screen-fixation, a body language
of sorts, you write back the way you used to call her, always with a mixed agenda:
(I'm sorry, but no umbrella modifiers make themselves available here).
The subtitles engage in an epic dialogue, the way the protagonists relate
in *Hiroshima, Mon Amour* out of sync with their lips and in delayed reaction
to their desires. Their desires portrayed in black-and-white film,
the only realistic medium for love and death, for pornography and ruination;
for the blanched complexion, the harnessed eyes, the bed-sheet toga,
the Asian profile as it smokes a cigarette and describes the mutilation outside
he surveys which time, to this day, is impotent to nullify.

"I simply miss him," confesses Peter Finch nondefensively in a tête-à-tête
with the camera at the end of *Sunday Bloody Sunday*, referring to the bisexual
dilettante in hiphuggers and turtleneck who not only tears apart like blood oranges
the hearts of both Finch and Glenda Jackson but has built a monstrous sculpture/
fountain in Finch's backyard which functions like a multitude of Water Piks.
His missing him strikes us as poignant precisely because this guy is such a twit,
memorable solely for a certain panache demonstrated in the replacing of a fuse.
After acting in one of the most famous movies in Schlesinger's career if not film
history, he disappears from future cinema completely. It's the commonality in Finch's
longing we identify with, detected beneath the indifferent features (ours & his);

the relinquishment in his eyes to outside forces offset by the surrealism
of a Berlitz 45, the fundamentals of learning Italian for the vacation planned
they'll never take together. In his decision to go alone we view the imperceptible
as if the shadow of a figure in the background, depicted in the generic male voice
who queries with forced emphasis Italian basics, i.e., What time is it?
The check, please; Where's the bathroom? Do you have Coca-Cola? What about 7–Up?
Appropriating the perfect soundtrack to the chronic nature of Finch's narrative.

All strategies fail by virtue of the effort to erect a strategy,
the desire to represent you which ends in that desire, incontrovertible
as the ground wherein you've been neutralized in a final democracy, hermetic
like a fantasy that exists for as long as it's made fail-safe from the real.
From the possibility of resolution, paradoxically, I want to preserve you.
It would be the only gesture that wouldn't be too late.
It would be the only gesture that wouldn't acquiesce to the East
and pay tribute, even if only in the secondary instance, an allegorical act
rather than symbolic, to its awful palingenesis.

A photograph of you finally arrived. "It won't be the picture you want,"
forewarned a friend. But how can one be forearmed to desolation
save by acquiescence (as if to the East), to its vortex, violet as the orifice
you'll never enter again like Russians into Prague,
like an Artaudian performance. Like Freud's reception of da Vinci's drawings
you inserted yourself, permanently, into my field of vision —
a field of moribund forsythia, a field of lake water, laminated like a frame
from a snuff film where the money shot translates itself into a death spasm;
and the lake, subsequently, translates itself into a kind of giant sarcophagus
where the heavens are forced to witness as if a suicide, unflinchingly,
your death in its varying degrees of deciduousness.

Our love was like the dining room scene in *The Miracle Worker*
where a young Anne Bancroft teaches an even younger Patty Duke to fold her napkin.
Our love was Helen Keller. Our love was Patty Duke. Our love was the napkin
finally folded in the end amidst the food-spattered, chair-broken dining room.

Our love was the underground stream, the water main, and the black lacquered pump.
Our love was the synoptic cognition connecting sign to signified in Helen's brain.

Our love was woodland before topiary revisionism, the person in perfect health
before the polio epidemic. Our love was over-referenced like this poem, a strip
of neon, the prescinded urban landscape of Venturi's *Learning from Las Vegas*.

A negative transcendental signifier exited itself then from category to extinction:
lip marks on a mirror; a trajectory within an eschatological menu;
a blackboard that foreshortens evenfall;
the arm of god cantilevered on the sky's counterfeit surface, a blur of flesh tones;
a love missive inscribed and therefore absorbed upon a palimpsest
like semen into bed sheets. The soul escheated to ash instead of air.

And real time, as it were, becomes impossible to measure as in Chantal Ackerman's
Jeanne Dielman, 23 Quai du Commerce, 1080 Bruxelles where the perfunctory preparation
of meatloaf becomes the simultaneous action of her prostitution.
The hour transgresses the essential demarcations of light and darkness,
a prostitute who does not look like a prostitute, which is to say a housewife;
the painting no longer defined by the frame, but by the *parergon*, the image
as a discursive grid, uncropped, detached and interminable.
The history of the frame reframes itself as the history of the failure to reframe.

The hour then deliquesces as the concept of the hour: oblivion contained
like an hourglass without sand, the sordid eye sockets of the dead
we supplement as the loved one gone as if into another time zone;
a barren prairie proliferated with winged monkeys and diminutive ballerinas
to which the initial prayer site was founded like a lean-to
both basic and fatuous, an indiscernible ritual of sightlining the horizon.
A nefarious face served as our compass, like the circumscribed appearance of, say,
the diamond ring X recalls on the way down in the elevator in *Dressed to Kill*
or a classic sitcom split-screen scene as in *Annie Hall*.
We moved toward land while drowning at sea, like Gericault's *The Raft of the Medusa*
(1819) where death and life intertwine as the labyrinthine structure of survival,
swine with twenty last breaths left inside the diamond mines of their lungs.
We swam until the absence became intolerable. The longing festered
and grew endogenously until our hand, spotted and varicose, let itself be guided
in tribute to human mimesis and the greatest biography ever written realized
an epoch at once open-ended and unto itself, a death of sorts like the death
of so-and-so wherein an ineffable part of ourselves died also;
for which we're still searching, counting the hours, red, blue, yellow, black:
(1 a.m.) the false panel that equals the secret chamber.
(2:00) the polylingual dictionary.
(3:00) the hour, on your knees, you gave to me, kissing my ass like a baby's forehead.
(4:00) pure as strychnine.
(5:00) the structure of implicit hope purloined from its antithetical nothing.
(6:00) you masturbating with a dog-eared 19th century novel laid open
across your chest, a punk performance art of open-heart surgery.

(7:00) the bed that never supersedes the womb, a futuresque casket.

(8:00) purblind thoughts, cuneiform writing forced into dialogue.

(9:00) the hour, a putrefaction of its antecedent.

(10:00) Concrete Blonde's "Bloodletting".

(11:00) pussywhipped by the phenomenon of time.

(12 noon) an amber contact lens.

(1 p.m.) the exponentially complex moment of diagnosis.

(2:00) the footnote to the hour (Columbia University Press, New York, N.Y.), p. 14.

(3:00) a pesto+parmesan cheese-encrusted plate in a sink.

(4:00) the demonstration of love expedited in the signifier "betrothal".

(5:00) the physical examination and/or the political interrogation.

(6:00) Paris in toto.

(7:00) the hour, on my knees, I gave to you, a ballsy, disembodied head.

(8:00) the phone call informing me that you are dead.

(9:00) the hours tied like limbs together until reduced to sobs and bartering.

(10:00) the Wagnerian week of your funeral in which blizzard conditions
flagellated whole cities, Chicago, Boston and New York, into a marshaled silence,
a hibiscus-like hiatus; stark; natty; a Basho haiku.

(11:00) Rudolf Schwarzkogler's *Action* (1965).

(Midnight) a discourse on pain that by virtue of its subject's inability to
be elucidated both continues and remains merely a discourse on pain.

We married each other in order to reminisce about hell like Dante and Virgil.
We were awed by the gym-bodies, fractions of ourselves who chewed away at our craft,
the arcane waters, black and portentous, cheap garb that lapped upon our epidermis
like underwear from Frederick's of Hollywood until we copulated greedily in the dinghy,
turned on by purgatory, both concept and reality. Later we remarked (crisply)
how like the Yugoslavian Riviera it was, cool and green in which the sea presented
the absolute as not just deportation from the worldly to the sublime, however
harsh, however billiard-bright in hue, however high-pressured the internal syllabus,
but intimate too, like the morning we made love in Prague.
When I turned my head arbitrarily toward the dormer window from the rotund ceiling
of your hairline, your face like a novena wafting upward in expiration
I caught a fever of snow descending as if without motion upon the rooftops
of Little Town, upon the tombstones that bespeak tombstones
in the inverted populace of the Jewish Cemetery, sequestered from the city
like indentured fangs, sharecropper scythes lassoed. And smoke, pink, turquoise,
ochre, lavender, charcoal, the reconstruction of history mutated
by the process of its reconstruction, extolled by stone chimneys, mixed inextricably
with snow, with your face, with the Yugoslavian Riviera, with Dante and Virgil's hell.

Like a wake we said goodbye to the body proper. With utter sanctity
we had the opportunity to represent ourselves in a single gesture,
dank, severe, insouciant. When I leaned over your waxen forehead
circumferenced with starched ruffles like a bonbon I gleaned my reflection
for a split second on the burnished surface (or was it projection?) for already
we had discarded ourselves as love objects left to be devoured like trespassers
pushed into a pool of piranhas. We speculated the way dictators do as entertainment
the torture of treason criminals, their public executions positing easy examples
for the *faux pas* of betrayal. We wanted to live off nothing, to eliminate
the factor of starvation, the unavoidable interplay of denigration and disease,
mental or physical, altogether. We wanted to regard, feckless
and arrogant, our lovelorn bodies hang like laundry, like Kiki Smith's, like
El Salvadorian civilians from a barn fence, putrid as dung in the torched meadow.

As witnesses to our desecration we are, in a manner of speaking, unmarred by it.
The road I walk on is always by a river, a river of water perspicuous
as plain English, its rocks like crucibles through which the river runs
with agonizing velocity, an almost slavish intensity, the sound of your stomach
digesting itself when you died. I walk forward but as if my back were turned,
the toothy spiral of my vertebra like razor wire capable of excising the world.
My desire, sore and swollen to a sweetheart pink like the feet of the homeless,
interfaces itself and speaks only in psychotic relation to the dirt,
pelleted with gravel and tar, your designated grave made ubiquitous now
the way a monk's sense of sacred ground be that upon which, wherever, he stands.
And the silence enswathes us like weather, like fluid, viscous as fetal fluid,
carnal like the electric currents between two replicants fucking in *Blade Runner*,
or a Jewish couple on the train to their death camp who fornicate before strangers
on metal and straw, damp with urine and menstrual blood and fresh feces.
Your great hands mash the filth into my hair as if into my brain when you come.
You murmur my name in its primal structure, solely made of vowels and consonants.
The silence pierces my womb. My lips swell maroon as hard, wild cherries.
I crawl down to taste our secretions in my mouth, a form of truth serum.
Silence, by its nature, defines us (and always will) as ensorcelled by silence.

The sky lowers itself like scaffolding, inch by inch, each day we're separated.
Soon it will press close to my face like the lid of my coffin, suffocating.
Unfortunately I look forward to that moment and find the thought comforting.
Unfortunately for you but not unfortunately for me.
The landscape, expunged of color, suffers regardless of its resilient topology.
My use for it damaged irreversibly by your death in that your death has replaced it.

I never saw you die so before me I envision you continually dying
a soldier shot in the leg wiggling like an agama amidst the frontline grasses
a teenager who drowns himself in the local lake at midnight
beneath a serene constellation. Taurus.
His acute longing disguised as a death wish sits inside me, just waiting.
What should be ameliorated only gets worse. O tell me, is death more even?

I never saw you die so before me I envision you continually dying;
the *mise-en-scène* of your dying I behold becomes, therefore, a *mise-en-abyme*
where before me wavers the apparition of the anadiplosis of your eyes closing,
like Mathew Brady's *Gathered for Burial at Antietam After the Battle of*
September 17, 1862 (1862) your body descends in the unending action of descension
like Caravaggio's *The Entombment of Christ* (1602) where the great, unself-conscious
arm drops manly and heavy like the arm of an atheist, palm upward as if to balance
the isosceles triangle that approximates the distance from earth to heaven, pyramid
point dead center, nail wounds which abound rubies and love but rest godforsaken.

Would I have preferred you to die in my arms as my lawyer did in the arms of his boy-
friend and take your last breath into my mouth like the egg-yolk scene in *Tampopo*?
The lovers sheathed in white, the color of mourning, lambasted against their libidinal
curve, silver trout upstreaming, in a low-ceilinged, plush-carpeted Tokyo hotel room.
When you gave that movie to me for Christmas you explained that it was in
acknowledgment of our many conversations about food & sex —
of which there had been none, I thought to myself; naught but the autonomous meals
where we ate and discussed, sometimes about us, sometimes about who-knows-what,
or the isolated sex acts where we consumed the other down to grist and marrow
like Goya's *Saturn Devouring One of His Children* (1820-23).
And I guess like Goya's *The Sleep of Reason Produces Monsters* (1798) our desire
infiltrated our Filofaxes as goblins do the blank tableau of a child's sexual fantasy,
our efforts to quarantine, to put to sleep the lynxes, accrued as failures
that metamorphosed in meaning as the human being does after gross anatomy.
So well acquainted with interiority, the blustery, bat-infested cave of it,
we stepped somnambulistically without footprints throughout its depths while sparrows
swandive for a larynx, spiders suspended like chandeliers metabolize our eyeballs
and rats gnaw on our toes rancid from cuts and blisters acquired from the miles hiked
we could no longer measure. To the extent to which we sought after the flesh,
paradoxically (and equanimously) we became impervious to it:
the orgasm, orbiting until obsolete as Old English; the voice dismantled
in the process of its articulation until it perennializes only as a myth of origin.

I want nothing now. My dreams extinguished by the weight of their prostration,
en masse in a dull, iridescent confliction like a migraine, or caucus of Greek widows
finagling amidst the butcher-knife precision of Athenian light in the agora.
My disappointment unhinges from its causality, inconsequential as their shrouds
as the shadows of great pines that pretend to guard.
It's a lie they're delicate. It's a lie they're transparent.
Their tresses impound your face, your decapitation discovered netted in seaweed —
the first of many: an underwater mass grave, a noyade that's fracas then tranquil.
I'm afraid to walk atop the trapped faces that refuse burial,
that address me in the *tu* form rather than the formal;
their hair which grows even after death weaves round, entangles my ankles.
Their attachment to the ground, to the ocean's surface, to life, to me
conspires as dense, complex, and judgmental. They persecute me incestuously.
They mock me when I brush my teeth. They poke me awake when I try to sleep.
They posit little clues that might lead to pleasure then erase them when I wake.

I want nothing now and therefore it's nothing that wants me
like the face of Sharon Tate and her reflection in the vanity-table mirror
when she watches herself overdose in *Valley of the Dolls*.
She regards the puzzle of black (her reflection) piecemeal its way out
of her cognition as she lies down on the purple crushed-velvet bedspread
and waits for all the pieces to break apart fully and fade away into a vacuous
mist of animated planets and stars, just like a night scene in *Fantasia*.

Death could vouchsafe itself as this beguiling, I contemplate from my camouflaged
prison outside the television screen: as a swatch of wings like a falling horse
that recovers itself, a pair of arms proved better suited than I to hold you.
It's what death deals out like spades and hearts in its trail which defines
the ruination, fragile smoking spirals after a firecracker's launch;
vestiges autumnal as dusk of the empty shirt, the faded jeans and cowboy boots
flail independently as if puppeteered in a dusk autumnal as vestiges of death.

"I feel love for no one," I reply robotically to a new friend over a side dish
of soba noodles, who's inquired after my progress on the all too familiar
bereavement schedule, having lost his lover seven months beforehand.
I deliver my statement flat as filed taxes and directly cruel since it includes
everybody, but he knows the brutality like a brisk shower will help revive me.
I rerun this scene in my head when I get home, sitting on the edge of any chair
as has become my habit lately, this sentiment of defiance especially highlighted:
a selection from Jenny Holzer's *Truisms* on Spectacolor Board, Times Square (1982).
The street traffic configures a sonant fugue, mediocre and listless.

The maple floors of my apartment gleam with the taupe astringency of twilight,
an unalloyed lucency which, as if inverse to the eternal flame,
erects a tribute to emptiness that must represent itself in emptiness.
The appropriate memoriam to your loss would be then the gesture that offers nothing
unable to be distinguished from cab flagging, a wrist wagging *au revoir*
or the finger fanning "fey" to communicate disgust. Hence every movement toward
the future becomes a method too of grief, each reflexed yawn when propped upright
on my beached futon in the morning, a mannered agony, a way of bringing you with me.

But the day overdetermined by your death blacks out like a Swedish winter.
No matter how eloquently Rousseauean, I rebel against its doctrine.
I study myself like a caged species from a fly's perspective in the corner,
my face, a dab of white, flame-like, that waxes and wanes, anorexic and quixotic,
my neck broken by the news that you've died, my eyes just holes where ants
already nest, my vest pelleted by tears that emit miraculously in their absence.
The darkness of the cell intensifies until it swells to a concentrated pitch
so hot it melts the paint which drips in a sheet putty gray as post-mortem flesh.
Clear vomit pours from my mouth like your cum, spring water spilled
into my Chinese red shit & piss bucket. The guards check me like a roast
and laugh at the sounds I make puking. Their voices echo like car alarms
louder than usual. The metal chute shunts, an amputation.

What could stop this torture except to join you?
What amputation would I be willing to undergo just to touch you again?
Yesterday when I received my 1994-95 NYNEX White Pages I checked immediately
to see that, sure enough, you'd mistakenly been relisted
and reveled momentarily in the delusion that I could call you.
But we are not, like California and New York, touching now.

I reach inside for the wild goose, a spot somatically deficient as scar tissue;
a soreness deep inside the solar plexus where the meat hook disengaged itself
just before death a long time ago. Like a Wordsworthian spot of time
it occludes my vision, the dark end of the spectrum equivalent to blindness.
It exists as freestanding in its darkness like Pluto in the galaxy
like the arcanum of your remains, at once bountiful and empty
a box, a perimeter, a cylinder, a silo, a corridor, a place I mentally point to
doubled over in a club chair on a schedule of Saturday morning crying jags,
a container wherein whatever we had (love would describe but a part of it)
circulates unto itself in self-memoriam, in lack of recourse as a recourse to lack,
a kind of John Cagean ode to Elisabeth Kubler-Ross' five phases of dying:
denial and isolation, anger, bargaining, depression, and acceptance.

The way a Ping-Pong ball stays suspended upon an air-jet, it perpetuates
for no reason save as an illustration of the phenomenon of perpetuation,
like listening to your voice preserved on old phone machine messages.

Our love is now a videotape of you interviewed five months before you died.
Our love is the muddle of landscape behind your macho pontifications
and somewhat effeminate gesticulations; our love is the pontifications
and gesticulations themselves, the sprig of chest hairs your half-open shirt
reveals, your mouth over the course of nine years and the evolution of its kiss
encountered like the kiss itself . . . anew.

Our love is now our love *passé*, both white and stained like a peace protest flag
wrung out of an Everyman's window. It ripples opaquely in early spring humidity
as if in demonstration to the futility of demonstrations.
Our love is the hangover of nausea when I'm forced to press "rewind".

Cinéma vérité recuperates reality in order to produce its fabrication
like a patient's slow readaptation to life when diagnosed with a terminal illness:
the abridged version we term "the present" sodomized by the overrated concept
of the moment, for no moment abides alone like an atypical cell, like a birch,
like a glass of undrinkable tap water. Moments adjoin us
as rope does rock climbers so that when you died I experienced asunder
the crashing weight against the nylon cradle which secures the pelvis,
a kind of metaphysical chastity belt. A twisted eroticism shot through my body,
a bizarre assimilation of the bygone way you entered me;
as if I had lowered you, leashed incrementally into the pit of your grave myself
and put you to bed for the last time, a boy giant
my calves bulging, my forearms irreversibly elongated maybe as much as 1/4˝.

Moments in the myriad of their congregation (the way molecules constitute us)
conspire like mountains or forests at the same time they feign fragility
until little moments succeed in sentimentalizing themselves into "mementos".
Memento! Set yourself afire before my eyes and you'll only further insure
your indelibility. Set yourself afire like Jan Palach
and endure in the architecture of John Heduk and the poetry of David Shapiro.
Set yourself afire like an arsonist's utopia, the spontaneous combustion of the world
that precipitates continually in matchbooks and sheets of notepaper set afire,
the grassroots memorial the inmates instigate for Da in *In the Name of the Father*.

Moments in their hokey mosaic of orderly non-order contrive a Zen bliss
Americanized as grunge mecca, a Keatsian ode that elocutes the destiny of Kurt Cobain.

When you died one calendar of disciplines became tantamount to another,
TM and shiatsu replaced the yuppie weekday that institutes
just another kind of suturing in order to employ a maintenance plan for suffering.
Good fortune or bad fortune, praypoems tied to twigs or executed
with technological grandioso and humility like Adrian Piper's installation
entitled *What it's Like, What it is #3* (1991) in MOMA's "Dislocations" show,
erects the narrative of the horse that runs away but cannot save itself.

When you died the skin was torn off me with a penknife but from no peccancy
of mine was this cruel procedure of premature shedding incurred.

When you died, the gods knew exactly what to plumb and pluck,
a garish sense of totality that matches my poetry, a mockery of their brainstorming,
the agonizing interims and recesses of conflicted juries that strive toward unison;
the invariable aerodynamics of migrating birds.

Memento! I am mesmerized by your tragic story, better than fiction,
better than cinema, yet distanced enough from me to qualify as entertainment
like the seven-hour-long *The Sorrow and the Pity.*

Memento! Larger than me and my dead love embraced until the decomposition
of his innards makes me faint and gag, but I stay, loyal and canine
afore your firelight where we lie, Adam and Eve, banned but gratified
for no longer do the simple principles of good and evil to us apply.

Memento! Your sad fate pumps away like the transplanted organ of an ape
inside the dying Neanderthal; the stilted diastole akin to kinetic sculpture,
Black Widow (1988) by Rebecca Horn. Black feathers swab my larynx, coax
me into a silence as an ultimate means for expressing ultimacy. I rub my nose
in the dirt of your afterlife. I valorize this abjection with nonstop tears,
with Kleenex wadded in my mouth to muffle the wails, another kind of kinetic art:
activist, unctuous, a confessional pantomime.

I adapt to the black widow that's replaced my liver. I let it break apart
the myth of somatic fusion which posits an anatomical model for the body:
the model for a bodily whole is in itself a fetishistic construct.
The model for a memory, a memento, is at once voluptuous and lifeless
as a garter belt, as a cock ring, as a dedication, as your spinebroken textbooks.

I will never be so happy as when you looked at me that now when I walk with
or without direction it's always into the invisible penetration of your stare.

I will never be so happy now that off foreign blood I must live, a black widow
that feeds on red tulips until the fate of red tulips becomes mine to seize,
gone the way of wildflowers that exemplify "wildness" when provided
as an eccentric garnish to salads in expensive macrobiotic restaurants.

Our story thus best preserves itself in the *haut gout* of its erasure
merciful as a living will it remains ongoing paradoxically in its closure.
It lies prostrate in pretend rigor mortis like Count Dracula,
while the rigorous daylight moves unforgivingly across the beige features,
a topology enshrined temporarily in salute to the collapsed interiority;
collapsed in order to keepsake itself like a secret, like a secret box
destroyed in order to protect it (similar to the spirit of your cremation).
History passes as history, like a bride clad in white, by virtue of its disguise
as in the case of the diary painstakingly updated then sacrificed
which serves as the superlative example of what actually happened between us.
Like Russia's red flag devoured by historical reformation
felled rather than ascended like banished stars or winding staircases
an entire mode of architecture flourished then failed, its buttresses and steeples
stained glass and organ-piped music, gargoyles carved out of rocks that vied as
counter-voodoo dolls as if in the effort to contrive, to manifest the vile
in us, we could exorcise it from ourselves and with it its signification.
Aye, like an antique veil dropped before us once we redefined the past simply
by proceeding forward with almost a whimsical absolution, holy water dabbed
like *eau de cologne* at the temples and wrists before entering a cathedral:
The hour = Donald Judd. The hour = the Pont Neuf. The hour = the memento.
Memento! Your postmodern tragedy desublimates our story appropriately,
a Baudrillardian essay on Streisand's nose vs. Barthes' on the face of Garbo.
Memento! Your impressive capacity for exsiccating time is enviable, ineluctable
as the phases of the moon, your beams achieve the mastery of laser surgery
where we, prisoners in our designated gender-specific correction houses,
correspond in the microscopic circumference of your light, our letters set afire
mere paper beneath such heat as if never having passed the censorship officials.
Memento! I place you alone like me, your kilned head bent on kilned knee
both more and less than a frame in this homegrown version of *cinéma vérité*
a lame attempt at the recuperation of reality by producing its fabrication and
with it the part of myself that died also but somehow surpassed the actual coffin.

Memento! I turn my ugly face to the anemic dawn: what hope once came from it
no longer comes. If given the choice I'd have gladly been the one.
There is no good last line for this poem.

III.

HIV, Mon Amour

HIV, Mon Amour

I.

Splayed fingers cover my eyes, fluttering, broken wings of small birds.
The companion poems of future and past lost from each other like birds
flown from the nest, the mayhem nest of my soul haphazardly thrown together
of pins and twigs, the last-minute contents as if last requests
of underwear, a clean shirt, journal, wallet, keys, passport, snapshot:
the burning cigarette that wafts in black and white beneath the blindfold.
They say you see your whole life before you in one instant
but what you see is your life as an instant, that leaf twitching, not close
nor distant, flaunts itself as your childhood from first memory until now.
Within the darkness of the blindfold sight veers blinkingly toward its extinction,
reverberations of light attempt to forestall the entropy of horizon from the sun;
in reminiscence, I hear shutters, swan-song white, from a house nearer by
slowly close out as if suffocating daylight with the only bedroom window.
And the dead child inside me disenfranchised from its burial ground
I'm forced to relinquish as a final offering to the omniscient threshold.

II.

The omniscient threshold, threadbare and glistening from your lack of pity,
looms with iron proficiency like the ocean in winter, cruel waves
that counter each other like Christian souls in a competition of suffering.
When life has become so precious you're afraid to touch it, the child saint
who miraculously never deteriorated but to kiss her would be her desecration.
It's this constant miracle that throws cold water on every conscious moment
like a slow but exculpated loss of sight as it ekes out a path of exile:
one puff of wind and tiny leaves alight all at once, future days and past,
confusing the air like snow flurries, the ground with a glinting mosaic
of immediacy, panic, peace, for which no amount of exposure acquires the taste.
The large shadows shift as if earth plates beneath me, recall my flirtation
snagged once again back into the undertow, the Gregorian beating of my heart.
When I say that I'm jealous of the dead, you turn away, partly in disgust
and partly in agony, for you can't provide for me what the dead know already.
My brain splits apart, hemispheres of apology and longing to be understood.

III.

I remember like bark my love for you bracketed above me, the ceilings of Trianon.
Their baroque spiritualism riddles throughout me as if my nervous system.
When they poured the cool oil dead center where I had been water-tortured
I flinched at first, almost convulsed with relief the way orgasm simultaneously
catapults you outside while hurling you deeper into the recesses of the physical.
I listened to my misery, now bygone, drip evenly, exactly as the water did.
O so slowly what tortured me today soothed me like a compress, like a cool drink
as if it were the water's destiny that changed in midstream instead of mine;
that cut the ropes in a fit of consciousness to ascend, a capsized boat, my life
where weighted down I had lived like Tithonus amidst silt, pike, and youth.
The memory, gilded, incorporated itself, a metal plate for the shattered brain.
It protects by deflecting, sun off a car roof, the possibility of loving again.
Eventually desire, so blanched from lack of exposure, will go entirely numb.
I fantasize about the takeover the way the bereaved begin to equate
death with heaven, their grief in absentia, sobbing with inexhaustible reunion.

IV.

From time to time, a reminder, you mock me, that there's no love I'm looking for
on the Formica-clean surface of the world. The windows remain closed season round.
Toward which view to meander, on which subject outside to focus, decides the optimism
or directs the darkness that effuses inside you, another view just like it
but distorted in its depiction, scaled to the size of your heart, larger than life,
thus barely containable: the lone birch, thumb length, formulates your spine;
a homeless person asleep under several layers atop a heating grate, the relentless
backdrop of your mind; the passersby of lovers or mothers glimpsed, objects of desire
as if through a peekaboo dress or see-through nightie, untouchable, torturing.
The attempt to caress, to mother yourself, adding milk to the steady bread and water
of your diet provides a pitiful substitute no supplementary discourse can deny.
I always seem to call you around dinnertime. I order out from the neighborhood
Japanese restaurant a dish called "Mother and Child." Once nibbled on, a baby doll,
then brutally discarded, that labyrinthine vernacular weirdly reinforces its locality
the way Chaucerian English continues as the dialect in the Appalachian mountains.

V.

Believe or believe not the moment of truth when it comes to you like the Gestapo.
The amethyst ending of day out the window seems as charming and holy as ever.
But the furniture shifts abruptly to smaller, the sterility of defamiliarization
replacing your home with found objects eerily maintained in arrangement.
Such a gesture of pity permitted per person acknowledges human vulnerability,
the way when admitted to prison one's allowed to keep a photograph of one's children.
It's the delineation of luxury versus necessity blurred for an individual second
(yours), that decides survival, i.e., toilets installed in more "civilized" nations.
Bulwark the world from its mercenary mission with sobs of pleading like dogs
whimpering behind the vaulted door. They've sensed the diminishment long before
the actual depletion of air. Forestall the sun its blinding glare when forced
to stare into it, into it, one day out of nowhere, you are, your head clamped,
eyelids stripped; refuse the painful depth with passion, unrequited, unconsummated,
for the gothic night. Our capacity for accommodation is formidable. Rely on it.
For swallowing at once the truth like a cyanide capsule makes suicide the only option.

VI.

Everything I write is dedicated to you though never publicly will I name you.
Eventually your voice, your face will fade like nothing I've ever known,
therefore not into nothing, but perhaps as a pervasive shading of your loss,
cast across my perception refocused forever in a way as to never forget you.
Few events indelibly change us, as opposed to influence, with landmark precision:
the near-fatal car accident that leaves you paralyzed, a blood test that reveals
a terminal illness, the blazing house where you watch your mother burn alive,
the death of a five-year-old child. Rarely does a relationship take on such import
unless it coincides or becomes one of these horrors, the factual litany shaved
down to the particular, the severity symbolized in a simple red ribbon worn.
Red ribbon tapes my mouth, blinds my eyes, erases my genitals, a censorship band.
Red ribbon strings me up, a carcass in an icebox. I furiously gnaw at the satin.
You were a witness. You too hated the ignorance. With you I could pretend
at least for two hours, I wasn't different. I'm sorry I put so much responsibility
in your arms like a five-year-old child whose life you could choose to save or not.

VII.

Will there ever be a point like a riptide that divides me from this fight
and delivers me as if in the wake of Mercury unto my dignity, contrived as courage,
the Captain that remains erect, though trembling, when he salutes the abyss
the heather-hued ocean that devours him and his ship and a hundred dependents.
Perhaps such face-saving gestures of protocol, once fail-safe, snapped and broke
in the course of trying, the last resort like retirement savings piled up,
gambling chips, on a long shot, a leap of faith where realization came in midair,
you'd never make it; the upshot of the great hand you sank your teeth into
and held on to, scrapping, ready to take it to the bitter end, even if bitterness
be the outcome, your skin gone gray with sweat, your hair, lanky and tremendous
in the past, cropped angrily almost to balding, your eyes ringed with exhaustion
exempt themselves from compassion, from cultural interests, from the peripheral
vision of human potential: family, community, enrichment; your stare set solely
on survival for so long, digesting metal, drinking urine, it's become albino.
You spit into the breathtakingly beautiful faces of the dead, enemy children.

VIII.

Enemy children, you yanked my baby away from me, her tiny fingers panicking,
grabbed clumps of my hair, the strands like red streamers amidst the blue mist
that rose up like spirits from the Blue Ridge Mountains, the cooling sun, a pitcher
of water poured onto them, coal pit in a sauna, turned up violently the volume
of her screaming. The sound waves still surround me, red streamers, "Mommy!"
"I think women who are HIV positive that have children are murderers, don't you?"
said the woman on a lawn chair as she applied sunscreen to her legs with a kind
of industry that now scares me. I looked to the swimming pool for alliance
but the green sheen from too many chemicals and lack of maintenance, made malevolent
its static condition, the patches of scum stagnating on the surface buzzed
in unison with the southern sun that forced itself into my face, an interrogation
light, until I broke like an egg into sobs and let out the secret as if vomiting.
The swimming pool, the kudzu, the lawns banded together in a lynching of green,
Republican homogeneity, that later so convinced I allowed them scrape me out,
a batter bowl. The operating lamp like the southern sun shone down with satisfaction.

IX.

Withhold from me like God the Almighty the antidote for this suffering, the cure,
a crystal vial glinting amidst the impartial clouds, a lightning bolt lifted
out of the context of its storm suspended, a snake-headed crosier ready to kill,
by scaring me to death, a slow death, with the potential to kill, but I will not
capitulate. I'll carry to the very top this net chock full of rocks, each larger
than myself, a hundred times my weight I'll teeter beneath, heave and ho the load
like a beloved, dying friend, my beloved, dying self. I'll drag my dislodged home
behind, climb aboard it like a broomstick and soar beyond the ultimates —
raised rails of a steeplechase, a field of poppies, lipstick-red and poisonous —
to the minuscule city, where the Chrysler Building in Manhattan, like a crystal
vial, pierces the razor-edged skyline in an effort to define it as vanishing point
of the ideal, cutthroat in ambition as an angel wing. Pluck a feather
from it and take it to this rope. File the wire knot to frizz, the fright wig
of what might have been, borrowed by the Devil like the coveted crown of thorns.
Transform the ring of pocketed posies to a laurel wreath or cut my throat instead.

X.

When you go you go alone, giving good head to a loaded gun. That's what we're afraid
of. From the git it's an ongoing love/hate rapport with that iron barrel, whether fed
from breast or bottle, operative always an ulterior agenda played like a music box in
the milky sky. Whether a spoon of nickel or silver, the moon shattered on the Aegean,
a bed of needles, a nude of marble, unstable and cryptic and of a rape mentality.
Whether the sex of the beloved, bending its back almost to agony over a kitchen table.
Its bound arms blur to plastic, its pawky ass rubberized within the myopia of
eroticism, fragmented like a page torn out of a porno magazine. The potentiality to
dismember your life, utterly, remains set to spring just an earshot away. You picture
the omnipotence amidst the black grasses of your unconscious ready to be revealed
like a lightshow. That desire will become confused with fear is what we're afraid of.
In dread of being terrorized one more time our desire will mount like a stallion.
At the point of climax we look up at the milky sky and pray for intervention. We open
our mouths, O-shaped like an angel's, lick our lips thoroughly as lubricant. Our eyes
roll back into their sorrel interior. Out of our exploding heads spurt feathers.

XI.

How to alchemize these feelings into love is what I pray for. Not before the cross
but before the icon, the denomination of Christianity etymologized down to a picture
frame, not unlike the soul's relationship to the skeleton, the skeleton's to its
decaying flesh, flesh purloined by mummy wraps, swaddling rhapsodized by coffin.
The cameoed faces of the Virgin and child float untethered like haloes, like passion
between lovers, from their bodies, armored by an overlay of embossed tin against
any potential skepticism that might spoil things. In a last rapprochement with God
you bend to kiss the glass that shields them yet again, insulated as a storm window.
The symbol, save for the stain of lip marks, atoned, rises invisible as monotheism
from polytheism, as Host from tap water, in the psychomachia of your brainless soul.
The two heads waver within the frequency of their relic status, like old Hollywood,
almost radioactive, split atoms whose proximity incurs a kind of tension that acts
both as a vacuum toward ascension and its repellant, a magnetic field of collective
sins in which your gesture, the ingenuous kiss, delineates like Azrael, like a Nazi
general when the train stops at Dachau, the evil (so much) in you from the good.

XII.

On the day the Virgin died the moon dragged its widow hump to the center of the sky.
It surveyed, glazed with grief, the scorched but august Grecian land it deeply loved.
The olive trees abused enough withdrew entirely into shadow, into negative space
that, like black holes, absorbs all space, detonator bombs planted in the darkest waters.
The sea swollen like a breast turgid with milk turned sour for the baby born dead
expressed its impotence in a stillness that refused to soothe neither man nor animal.
They perched along the rocks, adverted toward the waves as if to a short-wave radio.
They waited but the churlish wails like a lost dog never returned. Their brows
furrowed with sleeplessness. Their clothes camouflaged with dust scattered like dust
in the end, in piles of leafy ash as mutable and pitiful. They began to wander naked
as children. They began to invoke in each other, with their waiflike expressions,
a scavenger disposition. They panned the dirt for traces of the virgin, a lost ring,
torn lace from her slip, a buried tooth she had ceremonied herself. They suspected
one another as if, having kidnapped and eaten her whole, upon opening their mouths
she would reappear, shockingly youthful if not beguiling, winking seductively back.

XIII.

Despite our stupid cries (all mine), I gag my mouth with a handkerchief, the same
with which from the 747 I waved goodbye, the same I folded like an origami bird
into your gauntlet, the same I made a rudimentary sanitary napkin, the same doused
with "Joy" perfume to watch it tumble, autumnal and isolated, in front of no one
on the sidewalk for the hell of it. From this lavender zone you read as invisible
but sense the pinpricks of potential danger with an animal instinct devoid of human
intelligence, I allow the signal, stuff the handkerchief with coins and berries,
a potpourri for the mentally blind. I tell you I love you to mitigate the guilt,
I tell you I'm absolutely fine. I tell you I've learned a lot from this but after
ten years who can estimate what's been lost and what's been gained? I acknowledge
another winter alight on my calendar. I examine my body, a tarot spread for psychic
revelations. I renew my driver's license, receive announcements for the birth of
the second child. I live my life with my life ready inside me. At the gunshot
we'll spring, jackrabbits out of a briar patch, she and I. It's as if we created
each other as Mary Shelley did her superego in Dr. Frankenstein's beloved monster.

XIV.

Sometimes I step out of my suffering and stare at it, self-contained as a miscarriage.
I move toward myself as if aimlessly, a bottle tossed on the waves, in contrast
to the static figure finally put out of pain like a chloroformed body on the table.
I touch her glass-cold face with a glass-cold hand extended, a conduit for three
generations, the matrilineage of myself. I turn my aging grimace away from the sun
to regard, existentially displaced as a blurb, myself kneeling inside the pink sphere
of my recollection, both belittled and exploited on the dirt stage of its amphitheater.
No one was there as the beholder but us, when you lifted your face to mine with what
Diderot would call a "naive" expression of terror. The broken elevator slid another
twelve floors. The counter-day of fluorescence twitched on and off, mutating
all color unto the quality of black-and-white film the way ashes deliver themselves
to the wind. The forest shifts simply to darkness, barely gradational against
the sheen of an overcast sky. I acknowledge the white sheet that eventually covers
my head: black iris of a dark forest against the skull-and-crossbones white
of an overcast, marbled sky; my silhouette erased in the process of acknowledgment.

XV.

My silhouette erased in the process of acknowledgment, sepulchral and low budget.
Where X marks the spot place a poetry calendar like a powder-blue pillbox hat.
Watch the twilight turn, if only for an instant, the exact shade of ten milligrams
of Valium. It spews its blue-red blood thinned like paint, a vein cut to revive
the dying, running horse with oxygen until the fading flows all at once, buckets
poured, aquamarine and iridescent as antiseptic on the institutionalized floor
of the landscape. The pillbox hat floats onward into oblivion, bereft in motion
amidst the oceanlike corrugations. You say you pray for me three times a day!
Partly out of protocol and urgency to fill the awkward discrepancy of mentalities,
I thank you (profusely) for the favor. It may be the only way for one hubristic heart
to comfort another on the affront of annihilation, to pray, or at the very least,
to think of each other. These last threads, sticky and moonlit, that strap us down
to rock and tree and answering machine, posit the iconic pleasure, the overflowing
cup, toward which we grope, deaf and dumb, our crotches stinging with a woundedness
we cannot originate. Like aliens we rise out of nothing in order to return to nothing.

XVI.

The magenta dawn cracks apart the sky as if with a crowbar. Deep inside the chasm,
oozing like crude oil, breaks forth an unconditionality that never existed before.
Only in your dead heart did I ever know God. Only in memory, the baroque self-
assertive chamber of my heart. The blanched rubric of my skull surfaces, corpse in a
pond, root to offshoot of my face, free-floating at the top of my spine, a traitor's
head spiked on a stick. We glide beneath London Bridge, focused on the *trauerspiel*,
my future grave above, built like an Indian burial site, free-floating skull of a
cloud. A lightning rod splits the ceiling in half, loins of Mother Earth giving
birth to Perseus. Tears, spiraling in a single column, interrogate like an
ophthalmoscope of the Divine, or water main for atonement from a soulless source.
Please, show me what it's like, and take me like Heathcliff drawn in by the dragnet
of your cloud-white skin, your black, stormy hair; chest with shirt-torn-open appeal.
Teal turbulence of an ocean backdrop underscores the rolled sleeves of your forearms,
of great hands, as if making love, strangling my neck, in one painless, pleasureful
snap, in one jolt of passion, in one glimpse of lore-lorn green, aquiline mountains.

XVII.

If you know that you will die alone, like a coyote, like a Yugoslavian, then you
can do anything in life. The innocence of abyss arches its trajectory of deletion
across the image repertoire of your failures, mitigating the conjecture of tragedy
in the process, a processlessness that reads like a palindrome: matte white on glossy
white, white rose on sepia rose, the smoothed cascade of muscular infrastructure in
the marbled back of Rodin's mistress, the myopic teardrop to which we supply
the hermeneutic signified of "miserable". Your death floats always beside you, a kayak
stranded on the parched surface of the desert. Swaddled inside the *Todtenbaum* of your
negative future you break down like a particle, only the idea of which is fearful.
You guard your carcass, O papoose, that lies beneath the liturgical purple, blue tarp
of a lean–to flapping in a nebulous definition of fresh air, while underneath awaits
either a bed of nails or a bed of sweet william, the marriage bed you never consummated
but kept the repetition compulsion of excess and supposition going like some quartz
mechanism, hand between legs, nose pressed against the conundrum of your perception.
You wonder if it's worth the risk of slitting your wrists to shatter the glass. It is.

XVIII.

Down to the grave of wayward leaves, willful and idiomatic; a grave shallow, hence inexpensive but pebble-paved like a Japanese garden. Down from the shadows into the Ukrainian sun its regard devouring you in transport like Icarus. Down from a skeletal sky, fleshless and resentful, you've stared into their empty eye sockets for at least a century. Down as if lowered ruefully in a basket, Moses sent twirling and sobbing upon the currents. A peaceful breeze passes, a handkerchief, over my forehead. Down along the cliffs into the wading pool depth of ocean, released at random although from my prison cell I had not asked for a rehearsal. Down twelve or thirteen times the petite European car rolls over, the driver and passenger, two women, just friends, crash together in the exalt of a lovers' suicide pact. Your name uttered amidst all the sounds of your life ending, the instant, a sound rather than an image. The way a priest tied to a crucifix rushes over the waterfall into the water gutter cries out at the bypass to hell, from the underworld of his subsequent ascension to his maker; no matter the sign, the semiotic paradigm engraved in our unconscious reads identically, recuperates the same diet, the same deity, as if for milk when we cry out for mother.

XIX.

Unborn, undying, the corporeal foregrounds against its dematerialization, an ephemeral
monument to our pilgrimage. As sky painting offsets sky, silhouette/personae, given/
abstraction, orgasm/sexology, life span/eternal flame; so we come to know what's
incommensurable by the swanky, four-star, no-bones-about-it presentation of the tang-
ible, of the commensurable, i.e., if it's real it must be Memorex. The antenna of five
senses registers with the unilateral conviction of a single party vote. The carnal
chest pulsates amidst the corrosive solitude of the body until fainter the pulse,
until absorbed into the vacuum like floss my awareness cancels itself out; until unto
omission: unborn, undying. My face distorts "naturalistically", degraded by tears and
mucus, the forsythia of incessant hope. May I pass over effortlessly as an envelope
to the other world. May my breaths release themselves from a wailing mouth, carrier
pigeons en route; though now alone with a table and chair as I have been all my life,
may somewhere common folk matriculate out of the rubber room of a cold forest, their
hair arrayed with pine needles like sea life, their coats dusted with plastic, doily
flakes of snow, their arms, unborn, undying, outstretched in unison like a carousel.

XX.

Outstretched in unison like a carousel, bountiful and brutal and libertarian in their welcoming, the winter trees uphold an allegorical elegy to absence, an electric fence that grids, segregates the sky between you and it, antlers of caribou locked in defense. The profile of a caribou stamps itself upon the circumscribed anticipation, the commodity of your death, like Kennedy's embossed on the half-dollar. My name composed within a disseminating list as if it were from the phone book whence I came. The black wall of the Vietnam memorial, erected in the nation's capital, glints as if a sheet of water slid, a garter snake, eternally down it like a waterfall formulated originally, as it were, in hell. Black on black posits an omen, the 58,000 names of the dead soldiers and MIAs engraved on granite, black snakes in a garden. More people than soldiers in the Vietnam and Korean wars combined have died of AIDS as I move through the days of suspension, through doors or walls, powerful as a spirit, into the ochre room of my future hospice that drops like a phony noose in a spook house. In the pit I lie. Black snakes slither tighter around my body, naked as opposed to nude by their adornment, by their muscles utilized until they bring me to my death spasm.

XXI.

Opalescent, daylight fills the bedroom as water does a glass. Underwater, wrung from those bleary dreams, European police cars whisking through raindrench, potholes and interminable laundry, I come up as if for air but without the relief, as a sail inverts leeward to starboard, from hiatus to hiatus, noiselessly as an underwater ballerina within the matrix of her postures. Broken wings hover like the shadow of a branch, tender clouds that pass with cursory attention then mainly neglect. I stare back into the mirror of the anti-god I uphold in my disavowal, expansive and hueless, sheet metal which deflects as enigmatically the blank slate of my future, the way a shaft of sunlight, the first in three days, admits a useless symbol. The silence of the new year soon collapses beneath the arboreal umbrella structure of the Roman calendar. The tiny albatrosses renegotiate themselves into jewelry or paperweights, amulets honed from the hocked bones of Heloise and Abelard; locks from Christ's hippie head of hair. An image of heaven swings obliquely as atoll-like, *al fresco* but protected: tropical drinks, bandeau tops, stellar sunset. Alas a chandelier alights the flame-red antechamber. Mist rises in mifted ascent, humanesque as a ghost, cryptic as humans.

XXII.

A velvet pallor lends to my profile a waiflike, uncircumscribed beauty. Mitigated
within the context of my circumstance like a condensing puzzle (box within box)
I've grown conscious of the paltry, allegorical nature of my actions. Disenchanted
with intuition I've capitulated to method. Yea, I believed in Destiny until a
pregnant teenager decided to name her child after it. It's not enough to love, it's
not enough to work, it's not enough to pray. We must walk with the chiffon-thin
soles of our feet over the burning coals that expire as our earthen haven of clay.
What's destiny is to return to our primal interest in defecation. To survive a
massacre splits the self in half, discharging it to a wind-torn oasis. Erased are
all means of identification. Make a doll for me then, *faux* freak for its sister,
produced from a factory of freaks as if people really accepted you. Now there's a
puppet to survive me on the marginalia — but into its cloth eyes still sucks away,
ruining and vital, desire after desire until stripped down to the marrow, to basic
necessities; until carted off in a blue van, bound and gagged like a rape victim
like someone wants you dead. And you give me attitude about not being spiritual?

XXIII.

Why doesn't it help to be with people? Even the *brûlé* of winter branches conspires
against a winsome community. Perhaps the cubist cement jungle gym vacant of children
at this late hour reflects best with its brute honesty what's dry to the heart, hence
providing a kind of company: a state of things which both constricts and hollows out,
raked leaves heaped upon a makeshift grave; the tension of the soulful yet soulless
double agent always witnessing, a miserable child without an intellect always looking
forward to looking back. Like slowly going deaf, the silence caves in shovelfuls,
a sound-mix of bereavement and impartiality: sobbing, male and female, traffic on
the highway, the incantations of some religious authority, birds, the sandy thuds of
dirt impassively contributed to the burial process, the silence that reverberates each
time afterward as if echoing. And as if by virtue of the litany of soundless echoes,
like the mystery of that dead person's unlived future, extemporaneously composed as
the belated product, were its requiem — the way in African music a polyrhythm becomes
one of interlocking hearts. Nothing, not the winter trees reduced to underbrush at
this distance nor their moulin-like branches, so baleful, has conspired against you.

XXIV.

The anniversary of that night like a mass to ebony, the memory cropped by ether, by
the semen stains on your jeans and the computerized voice, albeit human, that totaled
like a roll call my blood counts sliding. Who peered with me over the ledge, auburn
steep, which matched my hair color, and watched the toy sled crash in elegy to sleigh
rides? I couldn't have been alone that night for too large mushroomed the alienation.
Deep into the ravine I stared as if with a speculum into the Gothic steeple of me
(I could even feel the suction action), and beheld like a wedding ring my reflection,
a torn piece of fabric, suspended in vitro, floating on a mirage of Lake Katrina:
the continual postponement of my rendezvous with suicide. Now I understand Blake's
delineation of the prolific and the devouring, the deluge of calendar dates, Monday
through Friday, qualified with asterisks, exclamations and dollar signs translated as
this revisionism perfected in retrospect like cosmetic surgery. I wave the swatch, a
mouchoir for sailors, watch it descend, and pin itself, a rock climber's fate against
what he obsessively visualized. I recognized his open eyes, his bleeding mouth ongoing
like menstruation. Stop glamorizing the eternal. It did not give me peace of mind.

XXV.

Like a slow but exculpated loss of sight the forces of redemption muscle up, a pulse
that monitors the grieving mind, sound–dot of dying felled to a monosyllabic screech,
great redwood within a forest of the metal box where your soul metastasized. In the
corridor, the nurses' rubber shoes whisk back and forth, a performance art: that which
is ongoing defamiliarized amidst that which is not. The sex organ for love, the brain,
turns in the corridor of the head once more, muscles up its unconscious reflex for the
fulfillment of a wish, pulses like the heart of a fetus or the impotent man in love.
Lo, the carnal image not fallow but defunct, embalmed in the repertoire of its desire.
Lo, the repertoire collapsed, a shot buck within the empty trunk of the head itself.
I've lost all respect for you but none of the desire, the metal box once an automobile
where in the back seat we fucked. No accident befell the little farmhouse caught up in
a crushing dream of wood and fire. The car implodes beneath the immortal hyacinth of
an April evening. Evening after evening, I conduct brain sex with the screen memory, a
masturbating voyeur who experiences real love only within the closed loop the icon
fetishized provides by both reassuring & underscoring the verisimilitude of his anxiety.

XXVI.

My death will not be the beginning of anything for you like a cloud that
formulates the heart of a storm. Perhaps you'll remember correctly, for once,
the inflections in my voice when confronted with the bare branches of winter
trees along Riverside Park. Perhaps the silence which throws their impoverishment
into high relief will pique a tenderness you displayed to me in the form of an
isolated incident like an FAO Schwartz Christmas showcase. But "but" as in butter,
as in buttress, as in butt-hole, lubricated and framed within the confines of your
unadulterated lust, your chest hair matted into a wreath of loss as if suspended
above the chest in tribute to your lost ability to generate human love,
in a position that neither descends nor climbs the burnished goat path to some
fabrication of god. Your tenderness erects itself as fraudulent in retrospect
like the simulation of life pumped into the upstart cadaver. Like oxygen depleted
from deflated lungs, the tenderness you exercised toward me has long gone in the
fragile collapsing of organs, muscles and bones, of my body consumed by heat inside
what bestows itself as life's most generic forum (after the womb), the crematorium.

XXVII.

For one moment more of your preservation, I extended to you a disembodied hand.
A bird forms itself from the origami sketch of its ideal that's my palm print.
I open my mouth and a bird's cry expedites all that I would say in its erasure:
the dog in us. You take me at night against a bush, without overture, without hope.
True to yourself, you're at my throat, my expression gone white, overfrequenced
with emotion, eclipsed by the finesse of your brutality, a pine forest subsumed by
forest fire. The negative ions cancel out their calming property, an oil spill in the
ocean. Despite the decay, I lean my head against your chest and listen to my love
entombed, plangent and impotent as the illusion of ocean in a conch. I'm shocked
by my devotion. I walk through fire, the cords are cut, my body removed from its
context. Untethered, I float, a corpse offered up as carrion on stilts to totem gods;
stretched out, a canvas, a salt lick, a virgin, for only a god would seduce a virgin
until she becomes a whore. The earth is littered with gods, O Lord. Birds feed off my
eyes. You hear them (remember, once my voice) and think of the dog in us. You write a
very short poem in your head, the first in years, unworthy of record you later decide.

XXVIII.

You are not alone like a coyote. You are not alone like the feral cactus beside him,
like the parched terrain beneath him, cracked but riveted, like the loveless
surveillance of the moon above him, or the horrible tearing sound of wind when he sleeps.
His sleep is not yours, although at midnight you wake to the horrible tearing sound, cry
out to the fabric, witness the literal stripping down of your life into bandages
and ties, rags and bandanas. You wade through them, a macabre kind of confetti, on the
way to the bathroom. You are not alone when you return to your bed, gray waterproof
laid askew on the parched terrain of your carpet, to the panoptic chambers of your
dreaming. In one cell you work harder, disciplined to expedience & clarity. In another
you're quarantined, left to the desultory discourse of your delirium. An observant
nurse clues in on a certain word repeated which becomes the enigmatic signifier for
your soul like "rosebud" in *Citizen Kane*. You are not alone when roll-called for the
quotidian showing of your face in the window. You are not alone turned toward the cold
bricks tonight, when you masturbate in silence like the night before, the very silence
so eroticized at this point that a momentary lull in the madhouse turns you on.

XXIX.

If Nietzsche called his pain a dog then I call my pain a desire, a creature who looks up at me from a bare mattress on a bare floor, a kind of dog, a kind of child. I feed her teaspoons of mollescent porridge, a mixture of homemade texts, newspaper reports, and saliva. Her emaciated body appears even thinner as her head pivots forward for another mouthful. When she sleeps I work the graveyard shift and watch over her fits and mews, and sometimes interfere by removing a blanket in effort to guide her through a kinder route. And though I feel no urge myself I talk to her of touch, the mention of which she responds to like a wife and capitulates, Method-acting with an absence she loves. I insert my fist deep into her throat, for how could I refuse? Her eyes close almost satisfactorily for once. Then the lovemaking proper begins: unswaddling slowly the limbs, calcium-white and hypersensitive; her hair webbed like Medusa's, a moraine of personal history, isolates the bust into pastiche of a bust where, upon the foam-rubber pillow, as if out of Medusa's head she gives birth to herself; her face an agglomerative space of frayed expression, pitched and penurious. Her mouth remains open: tapped into some infrahuman dimension where multiple orgasm continues uninterrupted.

XXX.

Whom can I hold accountable for these symptoms of devastation, these systems of
devastation? Force-fed by some unmaternal breast, breast milk contaminated with *E. coli*,
I nurse on air, a breathing fish beached in a low budget afterlife. The camera
focuses in on the face, the prolonged close-up serving as an interrogation of sorts
as if a narrative shot in real time would produce a facial soliloquy that ultimately
deauthenicates the voice; as if at my wit's end I would reach deep into my throat
like a porn star and offer up as evidence the clandestine, testimonial heart.
As if the pink muscle, blood-orange blue and swollen as a sex, would bring the
audience closer, assimilate an emotional close-up, to the personal truth of dying.
The origin, a seamless dream of dying in which the self-witnessing of the dreamer is
seamless. The origin, the state of Oregon I've never visited but sublimate a sense
of finality in its grasses to compensate for the unfathomability of their finality.
In other words, I can't imagine it; the personal truth I offer, the enforcement of
imagining, the oppression of that proximity, the smaller hand forced by the greater
upon the electric burner. The voice deauthenticated by the ineffable until voiceless.

XXXI.

There's no way out of the rubbed interior, the ceiling which dissipates into sky.
Left shelterless, what I witness without leaving my bed like virtual reality
conforms itself to my bedroom: mountain range, shining sea, the funeral wind
that demonstrates its mourning by circulating obsessively throughout the pines.
Even when I climb out of bed as if lifting myself up from the floor, I bear against
the roof of an opaque nothingness, a dense invisibility, the vanishing point of my
body's landscape, the avatar of my maker as it were. It flexes about like cyberspace.
Gloved and goggled I touch without touching the sentient experience of my death, the
black-on-black beauty, jet water against volcanic rock, ebony hairbrush atop asphalt,
text upon excoriated tableau, Steinway stranded on an empty stage, ash amidst ash,
a march for civil rights which arches obliquely like the ship of its history against
the partisan night. The Rothko room at the Tate. Closer to what beauty is in its
confusion, I assimilate a relationship for which I have no expectations, ambivalences,
or drives: a two-way mirror in which I see myself only in absence, but behind which
situates a presence, a prolonging, if not immortality: my appellate interiority.

XXXII.

There's no going back. I've fallen de facto through a leafy bower, a corridor of locked
doors like a stunt man. O that I could fast forward, dismiss my stand-in, cancel my
performance feigning a bad throat, write my way out of it to a profligacy that would
fulfill my misery quota and be done with it. But the dimensions of loneliness only
become more opaque like St. Lucy's Day, where amidst thickening darkness, the short-
ening days, an aisle of candles carried by young Lucys refuses to illuminate outside
their jurisdiction like shore lights viewed on a clear night across the Atlantic Ocean.
They demonstrate a solidarity with light from which, by some arbitrary law of de-
letion, I've been exempt. High above the houses, in a lifeguard's vacant chair, I
strain to thresh through as if optical muscles after a time of repeated straining, a
kind of weight training, might acquire the capacity that would force this descent to
open up on a desert vista burnished with sunshine. But the ambiguous menu remains
like a constellation of bereavement. I beg at random, bury at knell, send adrift
on a lake, toss down a cellar staircase a note of apology, an expensive watch, pence,
a ponytail cropped from my head like a whiskbroom, for who knows wherein power lurks?

XXXIII.

I will not be afraid of it. I want it to be afraid of me, to recoil back into its
cupboard, hideous troll, fatuous trollop of a sea nymph. Back into its corner,
its mattress, a buzzard's nest null of hydrodynamic current, a drink of water
I refuse to drink. I watch it fall. I have no compassion for the dreary, wry,
bourbon drinking, chain smoking, bulldog faced old woman, her single gray braid
pinned acrimoniously to the side of her head like a beret with a sea lion's
tusk appliqué. For decades she's worn a wombat's money belt and I want to ask her
"What's in it?" That's to say, was it worth it to live so long simply to end up
friendless and weak, your hateful attitude clearly accrued over years of mere
experience, was it? One-third her age but most likely closer to the morgue
than she, she wouldn't care and that's the benefit of wisdom I loathe with the
passion of youth I don't have time to temper. My convex world moves in, an
execution date, consolidating into a single suitcase. Only that which I can carry
am I allowed to bring with me in exodus from my life, the total sum I know from
its part, a cruel prescience; the seer of my skeleton before pared to actuality.

XXXIV.

The dowerless agenda of my daily life flickers like the first takes of a documentary, some shots overexposed until the figurative obliterates utterly into an abstract for which no feeling of the figurative can be abstracted. Others, banal candids that leave the viewer void of identifying capacity, reinforce an ongoing identity crisis, the mirror image broken down to a shattered arrangement, an essentiality from which you are estranged as viewer from frame, beholder from painting. At the crack of dawn, ceremoniously you're sent out with sacrificial intent in a dinghy without oars, onward into a lawless but meritorious terrain, forced to find the god within although you've already explained your atheism. So you make a god out of the image of your grave. You recognize the rectangle with sober regard as the undulating reflection of your face in the water. You worship it as if synthetic like a good capitalist. You fetishize the decapitated mind, in love with fleshless superiority. You demonstrate your love with a transferential bolt plunged deep into your groin. And no one understands this love but you and the Hemlock Club, your lips contriving a bastardized expression of mourning for the spiteful cock still inside you, a macabre homecoming to iodine sand.

XXXV.

Our love is gone like a dead father; HIV, *mon amour.* Our love decays, I regard
my father: a fly replaces his eye in the end. A fly now replaces my father's eye,
black and blank like the open grave of the sky, alveolate like a catacomb, a rotting
pine. My dead father rises in the lake, topside: our moribund love, his scaling
flesh, our love despite him, his matted hair that floats suspended from his life.
My love reframed by death fails to reframe my love like Malevich's *White on White.*
My body blocks the sun like a cloud underdistanced by an open grave, the fly under-
distanced by his eye. My body blocks the sun in a blatant act of necrophilia, my body
underdistanced by your death. I watch your face go black, then white. Into a cellar
we've been thrown on this earth. Even dead I love you with no diminishment, perceive
as handsome the ruination. HIV, *mon amour,* my rotting body blocks the sun to preserve
you one more moment but this loss is the loss of diminishment. HIV, *mon amour,* our
love rots like a pine, as a memory rots in the mind. What preserves our love is its
forgetting. I remember your voice but instead I hear a fly. To continue to love you
you must be gone from my mind like a dead father. In lieu of my love, Father, die.